DERMOSCOPY OF THE HAIR AND NAILS

DERMOSCOPY OF THE HAIR AND NAILS

SECOND EDITION

Edited by

ANTONELLA TOSTI, MD

Professor of Clinical Dermatology
Department of Dermatology and Cutaneous Surgery
University of Miami
Miami, Florida, USA

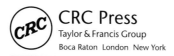

CRC Press
Taylor & Francis Group
Boca Raton London New York

CRC Press is an imprint of the
Taylor & Francis Group, an **informa** business

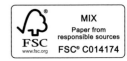

CRC Press
Taylor & Francis Group
6000 Broken Sound Parkway NW, Suite 300
Boca Raton, FL 33487-2742

© 2016 by Taylor & Francis Group, LLC
CRC Press is an imprint of Taylor & Francis Group, an Informa business

No claim to original U.S. Government works

Printed on acid-free paper
Version Date: 20150511

International Standard Book Number-13: 978-1-4822-3405-3 (Hardback)

Visit the Taylor & Francis Web site at
http://www.taylorandfrancis.com

and the CRC Press Web site at
http://www.crcpress.com

Contents

Preface

When my first book on the dermoscopy of hair and scalp disorders was published in 2007, only a few dermatologists were trained to utilize the dermatoscope for the diagnosis and follow-up of hair diseases. Things are different now as this technique is becoming more and more popular worldwide, with many articles published weekly in important journals. This book is much more than a new edition of my previous book, as all of the pictures are new and the content embraces nail dermoscopy and many hair disorders that were not included in the previous book.

I spent many hours a day for more than a year working on this book and want to dedicate it to my family, who are my biggest strength. Thank you Luca, Margherita, and Lorenzo for always supporting me, and even being happy to cross the ocean and come to Miami to start a new life!

I would like to acknowledge Agnese Canazza for her technical assistance.

Antonella Tosti
Department of Dermatology and Cutaneous Surgery
University of Miami, Florida

Editor

Dr. Antonella Tosti is professor of clinical dermatology at the Department of Dermatology and Cutaneous Surgery of the University of Miami, Florida.

She is worldwide recognized expert in hair and nail disorders, founding member and past president of the European Hair Research Society and member of the board of directors of the North American Research Society. Professor Antonella Tosti is the author of over 650 scientific publications.

Contributors

Francesco Lacarrubba
Dermatology Clinic
University of Catania
Catania, Italy

Giuseppe Micali
Dermatology Clinic
University of Catania
Catania, Italy

Fabia Scarampella
Studio Dermatologico Veterinario
Milano, Italy

Antonella Tosti
Department of Dermatology and Cutaneous Surgery
University of Miami
Coral Gables, Florida

Anna Elisa Verzì
Dermatology Clinic
University of Catania
Catania, Italy

Colombina Vincenzi
Department of Dermatology
University of Bologna
Bologna, Italy

Giordana Zanna
Studio Dermatologico Veterinario
Milano, Italy

1   Trichoscopy patterns

Colombina Vincenzi and Antonella Tosti

Hair and scalp dermoscopy, also known as "trichoscopy," is a very useful technique for the diagnosis and follow-up of numerous hair diseases. It is a rapid and noninvasive tool that permits us to recognize morphological structures that are not visible to the naked eye.

To better evaluate the hair and scalp dermoscopy images obtained from your patient, you have to familiarize yourself with the patterns that characterize different hair diseases.

This chapter describes the different patterns that can be observed at trichoscopy.

Box 1.1 Hair and Scalp Dermoscopic Patterns That Can Be Seen by Dermoscopy

- Follicular
- Interfollicular (epidermal, vascular, and pigment related)
- Hair shaft
- Hair roots through the scalp

FOLLICULAR PATTERNS

Box 1.2 Follicular Patterns

- Yellow dots
- Pinpoint white dots
- Red dots
- Blue–gray dots arranged in a target pattern
- Keratotic plugs
- Gray–white halos
- Peripilar signs
- Empty follicles
- Loss of follicular openings

Box 1.3 Yellow Dots (Figures 1.1 through 1.4)

- Yellow dots are round or polycyclic yellow to yellow–pink dots that can be seen at all magnifications.
- Yellow dots can be empty or contain vellus hairs or broken hair shafts.
- Yellow dots correspond to the dilated infundibular ostia filled with sebum and degenerated follicular keratinocytes.
- Yellow dots are typical of alopecia areata, but are also seen in alopecia areata incognito, severe androgenetic alopecia, trichotillomania, and chemotherapy alopecia.
- Yellow dots are visible in most Caucasian and Asian patients, but not in patients with dark phototypes.

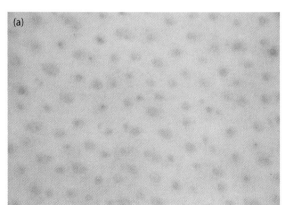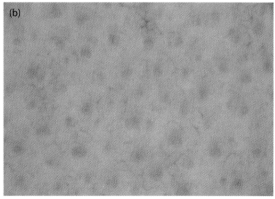

Figure 1.1 Yellow dots. 20× (a) 70× (b). Dots are round in shape and have different sizes.

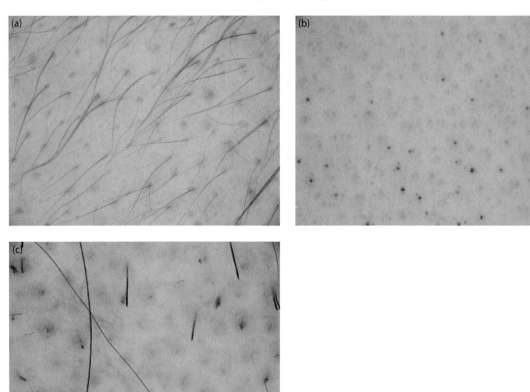

Figure 1.2 Yellow dots. They can contain miniaturized hairs (a), black dots (b), or broken hairs (c).

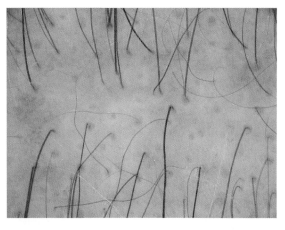

Figure 1.3 Androgenetic alopecia: yellow dots correspond to follicles with advanced miniaturization.

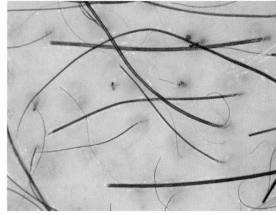

Figure 1.4 Trichotillomania: yellow dots usually contain broken hairs.

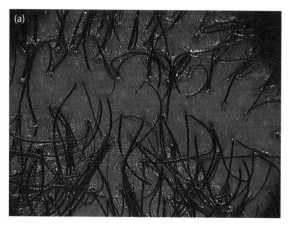
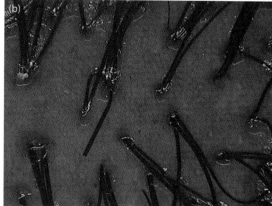

Figure 1.5 (a, b) Pinpoint white dots in the normal scalp.

Box 1.4 Pinpoint White Dots (Figures 1.5 through 1.7)

- Pinpoint white dots are characteristic of the black scalp.
- Pinpoint white dots are seen in the normal scalp interspersed between the hair follicles.
- Pinpoint white dots correspond to follicular and sweat glands openings.
- Pinpoint white dots are increased in number in all types of alopecias.
- In alopecia areata, they often contain broken hairs.
- In scarring alopecia, they are irregularly distributed and interspersed with white patches.

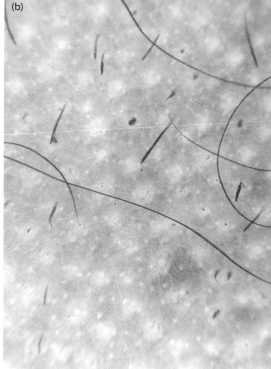

Figure 1.6 Pinpoint white dots in alopecia areata. They can be empty (a) or contain miniaturized hairs or broken hairs (b).

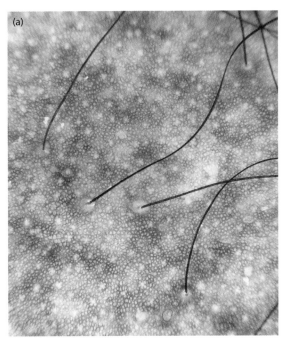 

Figure 1.7 (a, b) Pinpoint white dots in scarring alopecia. They are irregularly distributed and interspersed with white patches corresponding to areas of scarring.

Box 1.5 Red Dots (Figures 1.8 through 1.10)

- Red dots are a characteristic pattern of discoid lupus erythematosus.
- Red dots correspond to dilated follicular openings surrounded by dilated vessels.
- The presence of red dots indicates early acute disease and has been associated with the possibility of hair regrowth with treatment.

- Red dots are commonly seen in discoid lupus erythematosus in the black scalp when the scalp is hypopigmented; in this case, they are not associated with regrowth.
- Red dots have also been described in the scalp of albino subjects and in the glabella of patients with frontal fibrosing alopecia.

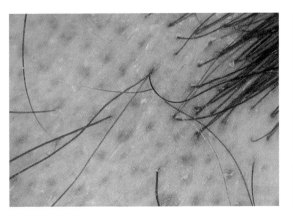 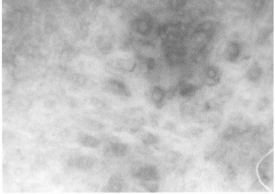

Figure 1.8 Red dots in discoid lupus.

Figure 1.9 Red dots in a black patient with discoid lupus erythematosus and scalp hypopigmentation.

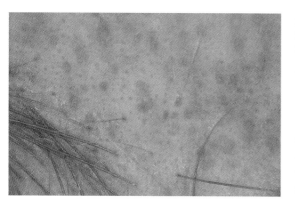

Figure 1.10 Glabellar red dots in frontal fibrosing alopecia.

Box 1.7 Keratotic Plugs (Figures 1.12 and 1.13)

- Keratotic plugs are a typical feature of discoid lupus erythematosus.
- They appear as keratotic masses plugging follicular ostia.
- Keratotic plugs correspond to hyperkeratosis and the plugging of follicular ostia by keratotic material.
- Isolated keratotic plugs filling enlarged follicular ostia are a feature of dissecting cellulitis.

Box 1.6 Blue–Gray Dots Arranged in a Target Pattern (Figure 1.11)

- Blue–gray dots arranged in a target pattern are a typical feature of lichen planopilaris in blacks.
- Blue–gray dots arranged in a target pattern correspond to melanophages in the papillary dermis and are a sign of pigmentary incontinence restricted to the follicular units.
- Blue–gray dots are seen at sites between the destroyed hair follicles.

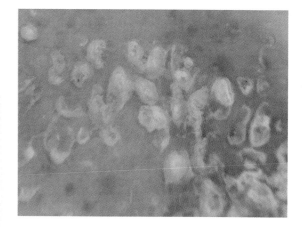

Figure 1.12 Keratotic plugs in discoid lupus erythematosus.

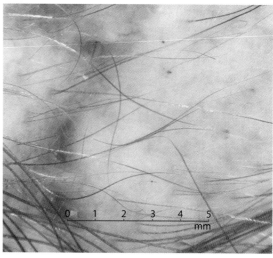

Figure 1.13 Large keratotic plug in dissecting cellulitis. Note other typical features, including scalp erythema and black dots.

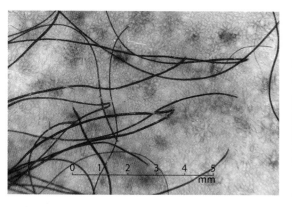

Figure 1.11 Blue–gray dots arranged in a target pattern.

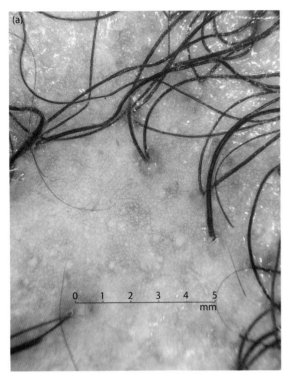

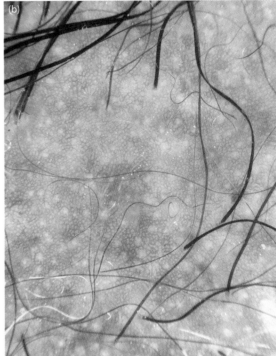

Figure 1.14 (a, b) Gray–white peripilar halos.

Box 1.8 Gray–White Peripilar Halos (Figure 1.14)

- Gray–white peripilar halos are a feature of central centrifugal cicatricial alopecia.
- They appear as a white-grayish circle of 0.3–0.5 mm in diameter surrounding a single hair or, more commonly, a group of two to three hairs emerging from the same ostium.

- Gray–white peripilar halos correspond to the outer root sheath of the affected follicles with the surrounding zone of lamellar perifollicular fibrosis.

Box 1.9 Peripilar Signs (Figure 1.15)

- Peripilar signs are feature seen in androgenetic alopecia, particularly in early androgenetic alopecia.
- They appear as brown depressed halos surrounding the follicular openings.

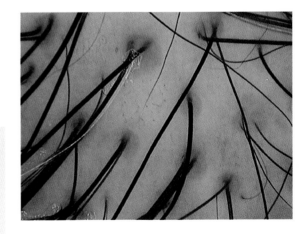

Figure 1.15 Peripilar signs.

Box 1.10 Empty Follicles (Figure 1.16)

- Empty follicles are seen in nonscarring alopecias, including androgenetic alopecia and telogen effluvium.
- They appear as empty follicular openings.

Box 1.11 Loss of Follicular Openings (Figure 1.17)

- Loss of follicular openings indicates scarring alopecia.
- This feature is common to all types of scarring alopecia.
- Other dermoscopic patterns are helpful for distinguishing the different types of scarring alopecia.

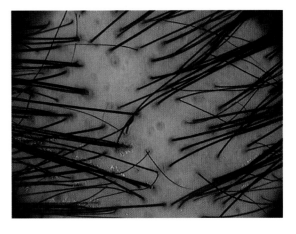

Figure 1.16 Empty follicles.

INTERFOLLICULAR PATTERNS

Box 1.12 Interfollicular Patterns

- Scales
  - Interfollicular
  - Peripilar casts
- Vessels
  - Simple red loops
- Arborizing vessels
- Twisted red loops
- Giant capillaries
- Honeycomb pigment
- White patches

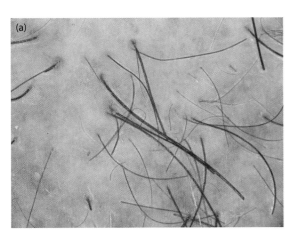

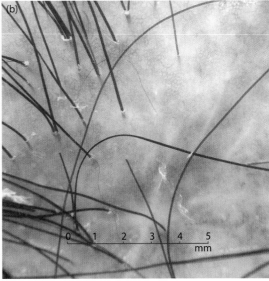

Figure 1.17 Loss of follicular openings in the white (a) and black scalp (b).

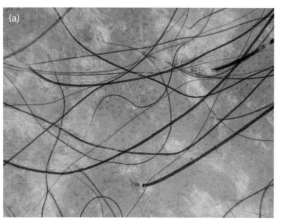
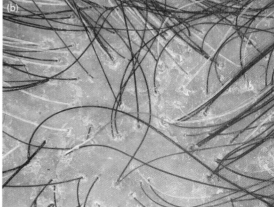

Figure 1.18 Interfollicular and perifollicular white scales in scalp psoriasis (a) and lichen planopilaris (b).

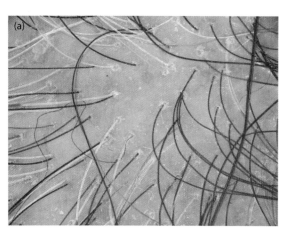
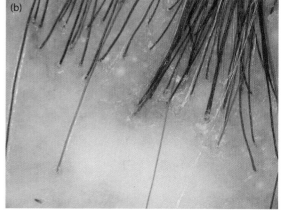

Figure 1.19 Peripilar scales in lichen planopilaris (a) and frontal fibrosing alopecia (b).

Box 1.13 Scales (Figures 1.18 through 1.21)

- Scales can be only appreciated with dry dermoscopy.
- Scales can affect the interfollicular scalp, the perifollicular scalp, or both.
- Interfollicular scales are a feature of psoriasis, seborrheic dermatitis, tinea capitis, folliculitis decalvans, and discoid lupus.
- Peripilar and perifollicular scales are seen in lichen planopilaris, frontal fibrosing alopecia, folliculitis decalvans, and discoid lupus.
- Scales surrounding the hair shaft (hair casts) are seen in traction alopecia, tinea capitis, psoriasis, and folliculitis decalvans.

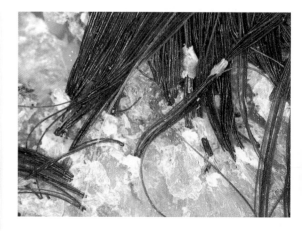

Figure 1.20 Diffuse and peripilar scales and hair casts in folliculitis decalvans.

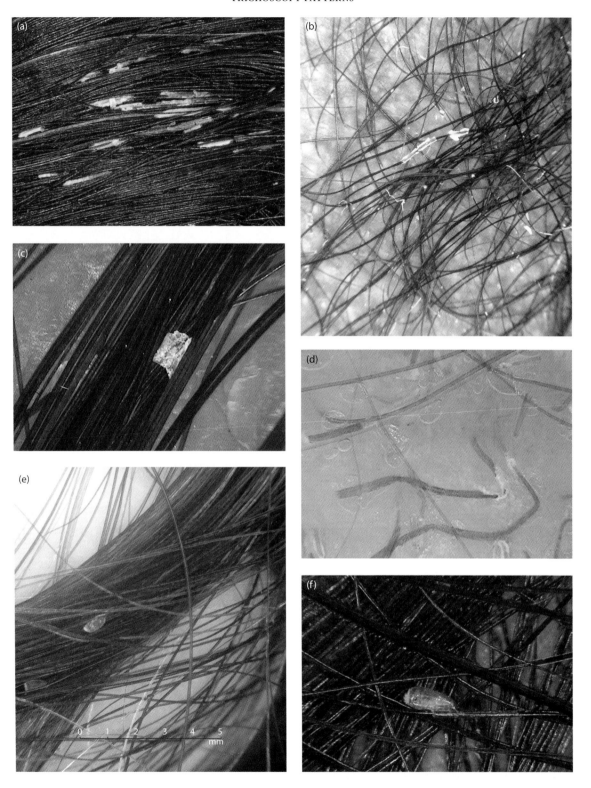

Figure 1.21 Hair casts: the shaft is surrounded by scales arranged in a cylindrical shape (a); hair casts surrounding a proximal hair shaft in traction alopecia (b); a white silvery hair cast in psoriasis (c); and a hair cast in tinea capitis (d). Do not confuse hair casts with nits, which have an oval shape and do not surround the shaft (e, f).

Box 1.14 Vessels (Figures 1.22 through 1.25)

- Vessels can be better appreciated when utilizing an interface solution.
- Simple red loops and arborizing vessels are seen in the normal scalp.
- Prominent arborizing vessels are a feature of seborrheic dermatitis and contact dermatitis.
- Twisted capillary loops are characteristic of psoriasis and are also seen in folliculitis decalvans.
- Giant enlarged capillaries are seen in connective tissue disorders.

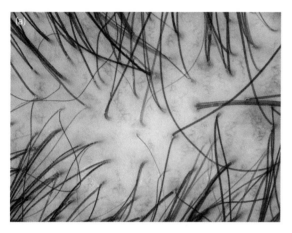
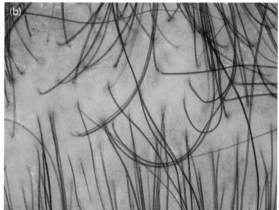

Figure 1.22 Prominent arborizing vessels in seborrheic dermatitis (a) and contact dermatitis (b).

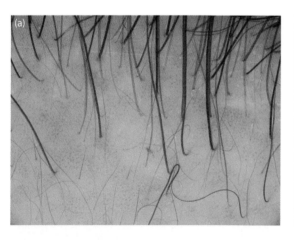
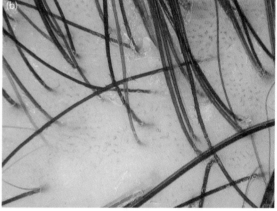

Figure 1.23 Scalp psoriasis: capillaries appear as red dots at low magnification (a) and twisted loops are easily visible at magnifications of 40× and above (b).

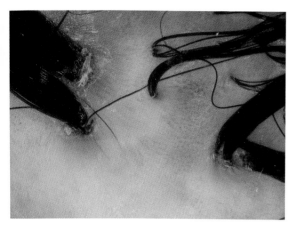

Figure 1.24 Twisted capillary loops in folliculitis decalvans.

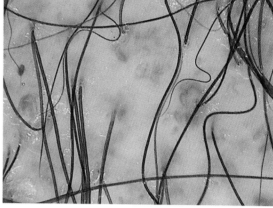

Figure 1.25 Giant capillaries in dermatomyositis.

Box 1.15 Honeycomb Pattern (Figures 1.26 and 1.27)

- This is a typical feature of the sun-exposed or pigmented scalp.
- It consists of a homogenous mosaic of contiguous, brown, regularly sized meshes encircling hypopigmented areas.
- The hyperchromic lines of this pattern correspond to the rete ridge melanocytes, whereas the hypochromic areas are due to the melanocytes residing in the suprapapillary epidermis.
- The honeycomb pattern is typically seen in the normal scalp and in nonscarring and scarring alopecias, except for discoid lupus erythematosus, where it is disrupted.

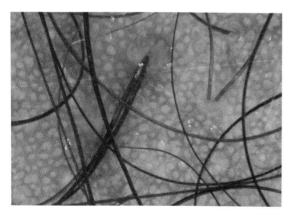

Figure 1.26 Honeycomb pattern in the black scalp.

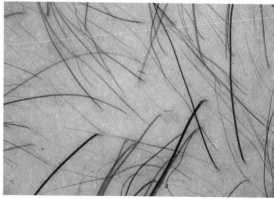

Figure 1.27 Honeycomb pattern in the sun-exposed scalp of a patient with androgenetic alopecia.

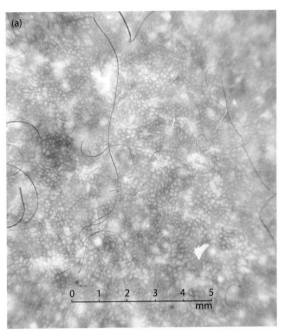
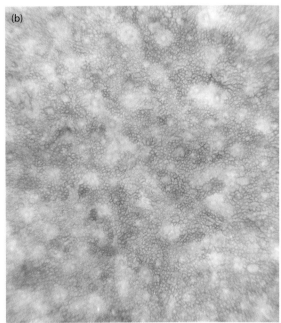

Figure 1.28 White patches in traction alopecia (a) and in frontal fibrosing alopecia (b).

Box 1.16 White Patches (Figure 1.28)

- White patches are a common feature in scarring alopecias in the pigmented scalp.
- They appear as irregular white areas devoid of hairs and follicular openings.
- They correspond to dermal fibrosis.

HAIR SHAFT

Box 1.17 Hair Shaft Features Seen in Hair Diseases

- Hair diameter diversity
- Short regrowing hairs
- Circle hairs
- Hair tufting
- Broken hair
  - Exclamation mark hairs
  - Caudability hairs
  - Broken hairs
  - Monilethrix-like hair
  - Cadaverized hairs or "black dots"
  - Question mark hairs
  - Comma hairs
  - Flame hairs
  - Corkscrew hairs

Box 1.18 Hair Diameter Diversity (Figures 1.29 and 1.30)

- Hair diameter diversity (anisotrichosis) is a typical feature of androgenetic alopecia.
- Diagnosis of androgenetic alopecia is indicated by more than 20% diversity in terms of hair shafts of different thicknesses.
- Hair diameter diversity corresponds to hair follicle miniaturization.
- Hair diameter diversity is also seen in alopecia areata, in which case the hair shafts are homogeneously miniaturized, however.

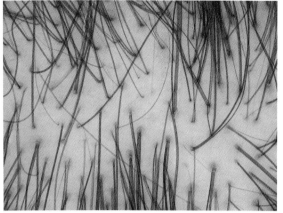

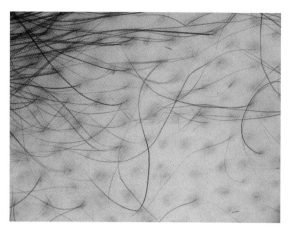

Figure 1.29 Hair diameter diversity in androgenetic alopecia. The hair shafts have different thicknesses.

Figure 1.30 Hair diameter diversity in alopecia areata. All thinned hairs have similar thicknesses.

Box 1.19 Short Regrowing Hairs (Figures 1.31 through 1.34)

- Short regrowing hairs may have a normal (>0.03 mm) or reduced thickness.
- Short regrowing hairs of normal thickness are seen in the normal scalp and in regrowing patches of alopecia areata, where they are clustered and in telogen effluvium, where they are interspersed with long terminal hairs.

- Thin short regrowing hairs are a feature of androgenetic alopecia and chronic alopecia areata.
- The presence of more than 10% or more than six thin short regrowing hairs in the frontal scalp at 20× magnification are criteria for diagnosing early female pattern hair loss.

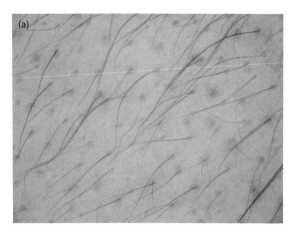

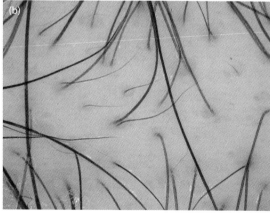

Figure 1.31 Short regrowing hairs of normal thickness in alopecia areata (a) and telogen effluvium (b).

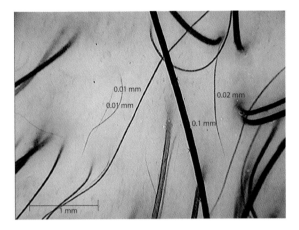

Figure 1.32 Thin short regrowing hairs. Note the different thicknesses below 0.03 mm.

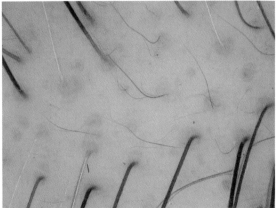

Figure 1.33 Thin regrowing hairs in androgenetic alopecia.

Box 1.20 Circle Hairs (Figures 1.35 and 1.36)

- Circle hairs appear as thin coiled hairs. They are also known as pigtail hairs.
- Circle hairs are seen in alopecia areata and androgenetic alopecia.
- The presence of a high number of coiled hairs is highly suggestive of alopecia areata.

Figure 1.34 Thin regrowing hairs in alopecia areata.

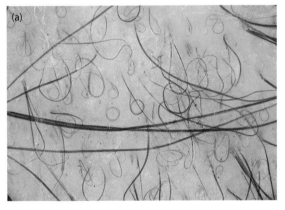

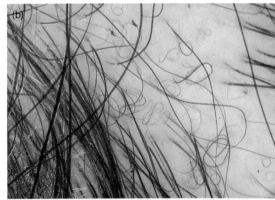

Figure 1.35 Circle hairs in alopecia areata. They may be the only feature (a), the prevalent trichoscopy pattern (b) or be associated with other typical signs (c). *(Continued)*

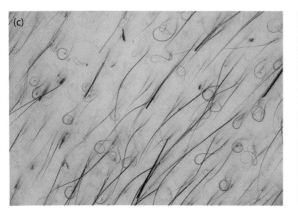

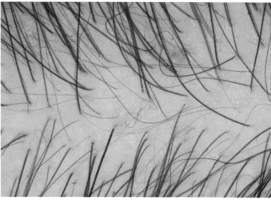

Figure 1.35 (*Continued*) Circle hairs in alopecia areata. They may be the only feature (a), the prevalent trichoscopy pattern (b) or be associated with other typical signs (c).

Figure 1.36 Circle hairs in androgenetic alopecia. Also note the hair diameter diversity.

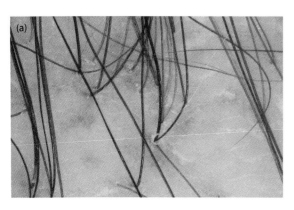

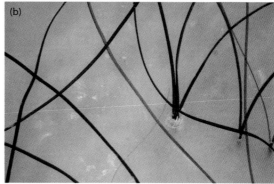

Figure 1.37 (a, b) Hair tufts in lichen planopilaris. Usually one or two tufts are seen in the examined area. They are formed by fewer than six hairs and are surrounded by peripilar casts.

Box 1.21 Hair Tufting (Figures 1.37 and 1.38)

- Hair tufting is a typical sign of scarring alopecia.
- Tufts are surrounded by peripilar casts.
- The presence of more than six hairs suggests a diagnosis of folliculitis decalvans.

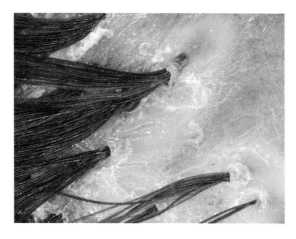

Figure 1.38 Hair tufts in folliculitis decalvans. Multiple tufts are present. The tufts contain more than six hairs and are surrounded by a collarette of concentrically arranged scales.

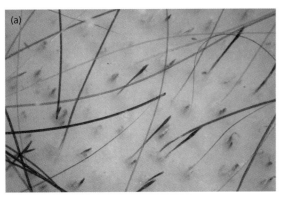
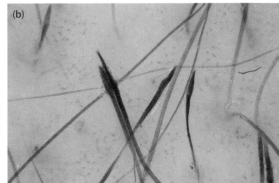

Figure 1.39 (a, b) Exclamation mark hairs.

Box 1.22 Exclamation Mark Hair (Figure 1.39)

- Exclamation mark hair is a broken hair with a dark, frayed, thick tip.
- Its proximal portion is thin and hypopigmented.
- Exclamation mark hairs correspond to telogen hair with a broken tip.
- Exclamation mark hairs are typical of alopecia areata.
- Exclamation mark hairs are also seen in chemotherapy-induced alopecia.

Box 1.23 Caudability Hair (Figure 1.40)

- Caudability hair is a hair of normal length with a narrowing in its proximal portion.
- It is typical of alopecia areata, in which is usually found at the periphery of enlarging patches.

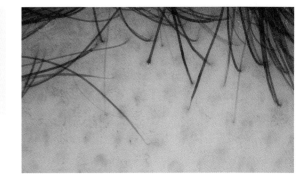

Figure 1.40 Caudability hairs.

Box 1.24 Broken Hairs (Figures 1.41 through 1.43)

- Broken hairs are hair shafts that are fractured at different levels from scalp emergence.
- They are a prominent pattern of several nonscarring alopecias, including alopecia areata, chemotherapy alopecia, tinea capitis, and trichotillomania.
- A few broken hairs are commonly seen in scarring alopecias.

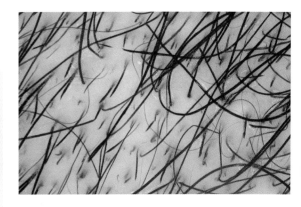

Figure 1.41 Broken hairs of various lengths in alopecia areata.

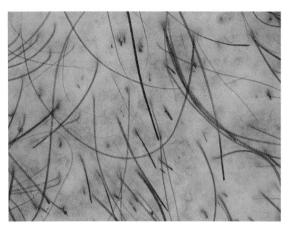

Figure 1.42 Broken hairs of various lengths in trichotillomania.

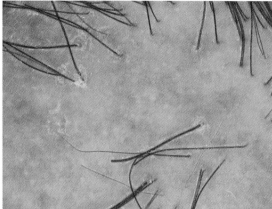

Figure 1.43 Broken hairs surrounded by a peripilar cast in lichen planopilaris.

Box 1.25 Monilethrix-Like Hairs (Figure 1.44)

- Monilethrix-like hairs are hair shafts presenting irregular narrowing.
- Breakage can occur at the site of narrowing.
- They are seen in alopecia areata.

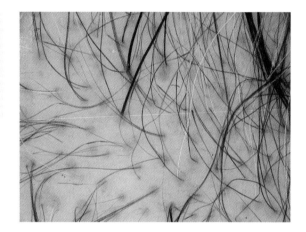

Figure 1.44 Monilethrix-like hairs in alopecia areata.

Box 1.26 Black Dots (Figures 1.45 through 1.47)

- Black dots are fragments of hairs broken before scalp emergence.
- They appear as black dots filling the follicular ostium.
- They are seen in nonscarring alopecias, including alopecia areata, chemotherapy-induced alopecia, dissecting cellulitis, tinea capitis, and trichotillomania, in which they are usually numerous.
- A few isolated black dots are common in scarring alopecias, particularly lichen planopilaris and frontal fibrosing alopecia.

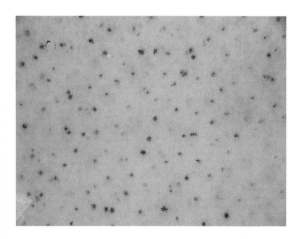

Figure 1.45 Black dots in alopecia areata. The presence of numerous, regularly distributed black dots is diagnostic.

17

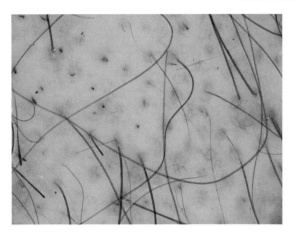

Figure 1.46 Black dots in trichotillomania.

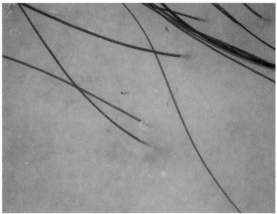

Figure 1.47 Isolated black dots in the scarring alopecia, frontal fibrosing alopecia.

Box 1.27 Question Mark Hair (Figure 1.48)

- Question mark hair is a short hair with a coiled thin tip, resembling a question mark.
- Question mark hair is seen in trichotillomania.

Box 1.28 Flame Hairs (Figure 1.49)

- Flame hairs are wavy, cone-shaped hair residues resembling a flame.
- Flame hairs are seen in many nonscarring alopecias, including alopecia areata, chemotherapy alopecia, radiation alopecia, and trichotillomania.
- Flame hairs correspond to pigmented casts at pathology.

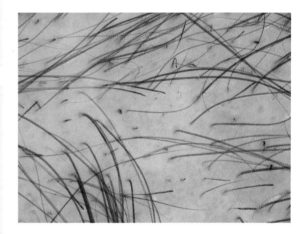

Figure 1.48 Question mark hair in trichotillomania.

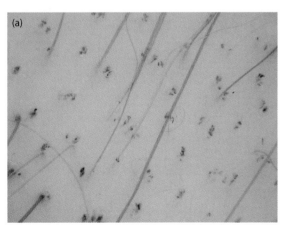

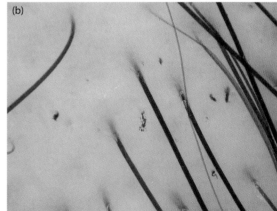

Figure 1.49 Flame hair in alopecia areata (a, b), in chemotherapy-induced alopecia (c) and in trichotillomania (d).

(*Continued*)

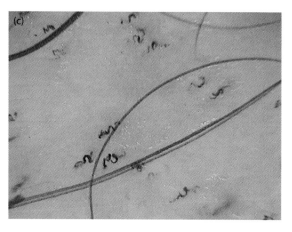

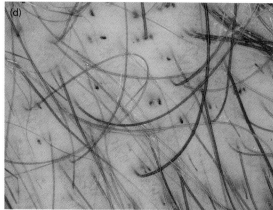

Figure 1.49 (Continued) Flame hair in alopecia areata (a, b), in chemotherapy-induced alopecia (c) and in trichotillomania (d).

Box 1.29 Comma Hair

- Comma hair is a short broken hair that is bent, resembling a comma.
- Comma hair is typical in tinea capitis.
- Comma hair is seen both in endothrix and ectothrix infections.
- Comma hair is seen in patients of all ethnicities.

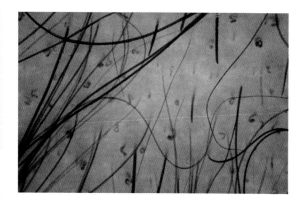

Figure 1.50 Comma and corkscrew hairs in tinea capitis.

Box 1.30 Corkscrew Hair (Figure 1.50)

- Corkscrew hair is a spiralized broken hair that resembles a corkscrew.
- Corkscrew hair is seen in tinea capitis in association with comma hairs.
- Corkscrew hair is seen both in endothrix and ectothrix infections.
- Corkscrew hair is only seen in patients of African descent.
- Its corkscrew shape is due to the helical shape of African hair.

HAIR ROOTS THROUGH THE SCALP

Box 1.31 Hair Roots through the Scalp (Figure 1.51)

- Scalp atrophy due to steroids
- Aplasia cutis congenita
- Erosive pustulosis of the scalp

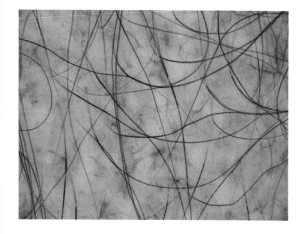

Figure 1.51 Atrophic scalp in a patient who has been applying steroids for many years. Note the anagen roots that are visible through the scalp.

SUGGESTED READINGS

Inui S. Trichoscopy for common hair loss diseases: Algorithmic method for diagnosis. *J Dermatol.* 2011 Jan;38(1):71–5.

Kowalska-Oledzka E, Slowinska M, Rakowska A, Czuwara J, Sicinska J, Olszewska M, Rudnicka L. "Black dots" seen under trichoscopy are not specific for alopecia areata. *Clin Exp Dermatol.* 2012 Aug;37(6):615–9.

Lencastre A, Tosti A. Role of trichoscopy in children's scalp and hair disorders. *Pediatr Dermatol.* 2013 Nov–Dec;30(6):674–82.

Miteva M, Tosti A. Hair and scalp dermatoscopy. *J Am Acad Dermatol.* 2012 Nov;67(5):1040–8.

Mubki T, Rudnicka L, Olszewska M, Shapiro J. Evaluation and diagnosis of the hair loss patient: Part II. Trichoscopic and laboratory evaluations. *J Am Acad Dermatol.* 2014 Sep;71(3):431.e1–431.e11

Pinheiro AM, Lobato LA, Varella TC. Dermoscopy findings in tinea capitis: Case report and literature review. *An Bras Dermatol.* 2012 Mar–Apr;87(2):313–4.

Ross EK, Vincenzi C, Tosti A. Videodermoscopy in the evaluation of hair and scalp disorders. *J Am Acad Dermatol.* 2006 Nov;55(5):799–806.

Rudnicka L, Olszewska M, Rakowska A, Kowalska-Oledzka E, Slowinska M. Trichoscopy: A new method for diagnosing hair loss. *J Drugs Dermatol.* 2008 Jul;7(7):651–4.

Rudnicka L, Olszewska M, Rakowska A, Slowinska M. Trichoscopy update 2011. *J Dermatol Case Rep.* 2011 Dec;5(4):82–8.

Torres F, Tosti A. Trichoscopy: An update. *G Ital Dermatol Venereol.* 2014 Feb;149(1):83–91.

Tosti A, Torres F. Dermoscopy in the diagnosis of hair and scalp disorders. *Actas Dermosifiliogr.* 2009 Nov; 100(Suppl 1):114–9.

Wallace MP, de Berker DA. Hair diagnoses and signs: The use of dermatoscopy. *Clin Exp Dermatol.* 2010 Jan;35(1):41–6.

Yin NC, Tosti A. A systematic approach to Afro-textured hair disorders: Dermatoscopy and when to biopsy. *Dermatol Clin.* 2014 Apr;32(2):145–51.

Zalaudek I, Argenziano G. Images in clinical medicine. Dermoscopy of nits and pseudonits. *N Engl J Med.* 2012 Nov;367(18):1741.

2 Normal scalp
Antonella Tosti

In the healthy scalp, the hair follicles are grouped in follicular units and are seen at dermoscopy as groups of two to three hair shafts coming out of the same follicular ostium. Follicular units composed of only one shaft are also seen, and their number increases with aging or hair disorders.

Normal scalp vessels include interfollicular simple red loops and arborizing red lines. Vessels are best seen with videodermoscopy using the epiluminescent mode of operation. Firm direct pressure (diascopy) on the vessels results in blanching.

Interfollicular simple red loops are multiple fine, red, hairpin-shaped structures that are regularly spaced. They correspond to the capillaries in the dermal papillae. Optimal viewing is at 50× or higher magnification with the camera probe angled tangentially. When viewed from above, they appear as pinpoint pale red dots. Their distribution can be patchy or diffuse.

Arborizing red lines are vessels of a larger caliber that correspond to the subpapillary vascular plexus. With tangential viewing, they are seen to underlie and articulate with loops to a variable degree in the normal scalp and diseased scalp of all etiologies. They are best viewed at magnifications of 20× or higher. This pattern is usually focal and more evident on the occipital scalp.

Dirty dots are a normal finding in the scalp of prepuberal children. Dirty dots represent environmental particles and are easily removed after shampooing.

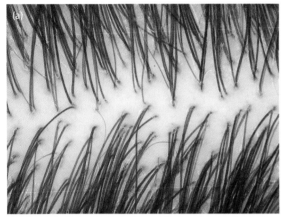

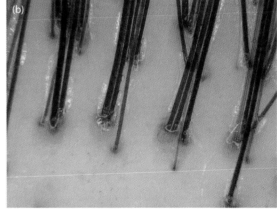

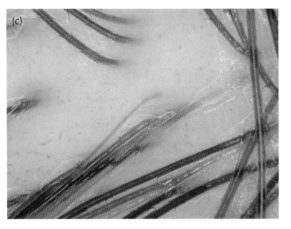

Figure 2.1 Normal white scalp. Most follicular units are composed of two to three hairs (a, b). Note the medulla, appearing as a white band within the shaft, which may be irregularly interrupted (c).

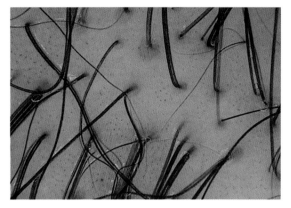

Figure 2.2 Interfollicular simple red loops.

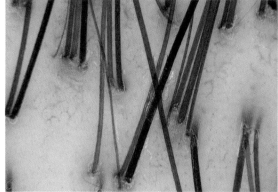

Figure 2.3 Arborizing red lines.

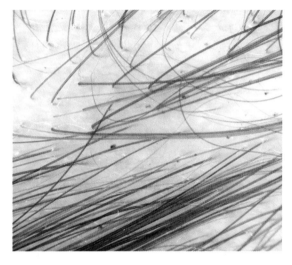

Figure 2.4 Dirty dots on the scalp of a child.

NORMAL BLACK SCALP

Box 2.2 Normal Black Scalp (Figures 2.5 through 2.11)

- Honeycomb-like pigmented network.
- Pinpoint white dots.
- Hairs mostly emerge in groups of twos.

At dermoscopy, the color of the scalp can vary from light brown to black and often does not correlate with the skin color. The whole scalp shows a honeycomb-like pigmented network characterized by pigmented lines corresponding to rete ridge melanocytes, which surround hypochromic areas. Perifollicular and interfollicular

erythema is also common, but the sizes and shapes of vessels are not easily seen.

A unique feature of the pigmented scalp is the presence of pinpoint white dots, which are small (0.2–0.3 mm) white dots that are regularly distributed between the follicular units. These dots correspond to sweat gland openings and empty follicular openings, and their number considerably increases in all types of alopecia.

Hair density in people of African descent is lower than in Caucasians and the follicular units most commonly consist of a couple of hairs emerging together. Single hairs and groups of three hairs are also seen. The hair shafts have a flattened shape and show irregular torsions. The hair shafts that are extracted with the pull or the tug test frequently present knots and fissures.

The scalp often presents scales and small particles that correspond to residues of leave-on products.

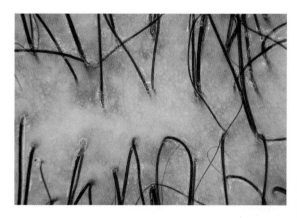

Figure 2.5 Honeycomb pigmented network. A homogeneous mosaic of contiguous rings characterized by a central hypopigmented area surrounded by a grid of pigmented lines.

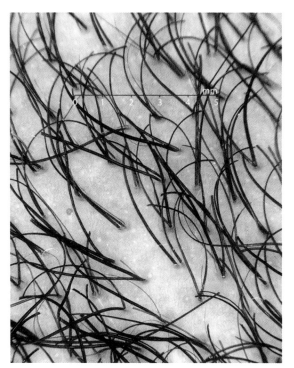

Figure 2.6 Most follicular units consist of two hairs.

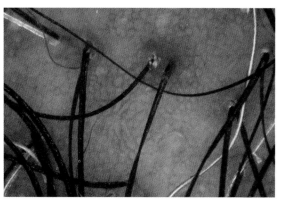

Figure 2.7 Hair shafts with a flattened shape and showing irregular torsions.

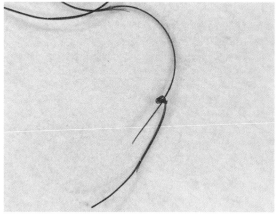

Figure 2.8 Dermoscopy of a "shed" hair showing knots and fissures.

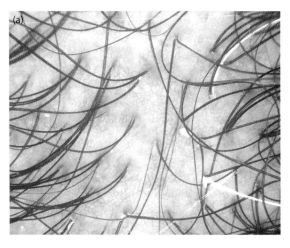

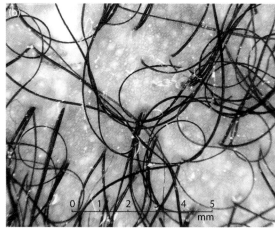

Figure 2.9 (a, b) The normal scalp often shows erythema, but the pigmented network does not allow for visualizing vascular patterns. Also note the presence of product residues (b).

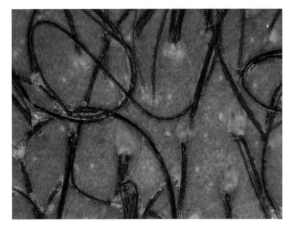

Figure 2.10 Pinpoint white dots.

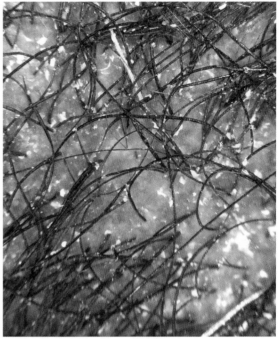

Figure 2.11 The scalp frequently presents scales and residues of products that are utilized to style the hair and moisturize the scalp.

SUGGESTED READINGS

Abraham LS, Piñeiro-Maceira J, Duque-Estrada B, Barcaui CB, Sodré CT. Pinpoint white dots in the scalp: Dermoscopic and histopathologic correlation. *J Am Acad Dermatol.* 2010 Oct;63(4):721–2.

Fu JM, Starace M, Tosti A. A new dermoscopic finding in healthy children. *Arch Dermatol.* 2009 May; 145(5):596–7.

Miteva M, Tosti A. Hair and scalp dermatoscopy. *J Am Acad Dermatol.* 2012 Nov;67(5):1040–8.

Rakowska A. Trichoscopy (hair and scalp videodermoscopy) in the healthy female. Method standardization and norms for measurable parameters. *J Dermatol Case Rep.* 2009 Apr;3(1):14–9.

Ross EK, Vincenzi C, Tosti A. Videodermoscopy in the evaluation of hair and scalp disorders. *J Am Acad Dermatol.* 2006 Nov;55(5):799–806.

Yin NC, Tosti A. A systematic approach to Afro-textured hair disorders: Dermatoscopy and when to biopsy. *Dermatol Clin.* 2014 Apr;32(2):145–51.

3 Instruments for scalp dermoscopy
Colombina Vincenzi and Antonella Tosti

Scalp dermoscopy (also known as trichoscopy) is the examination of the scalp with a dermatoscope. This traditionally consists of a magnifier (typically 10×), a non-polarized light source, a transparent plate, and a liquid medium between the instrument and the scalp. Modern dermatoscopes use polarized light instead of a liquid medium in order to eliminate skin surface reflections.

Some instruments, such as the digital epiluminescence dermatoscopes, digitally capture and process the images. Digital dermatoscopy offers the advantage of storing the images such that they can be compared with those obtained during the patient's next visit, which is very important in the case of hair disorders.

Instruments for digital dermatoscopy reach magnifications ranging from 20× to 1000×. Most studies on scalp dermoscopy have been conducted with magnifications ranging from 20× to 70×. Instruments can also be equipped with software to measure relevant trichological parameters (FotoFinder Trichoscale).

> *Box 3.1* Instruments for Scalp Dermoscopy (Figure 3.1)
>
> - Handyscope®
> - Veox DermScope®
> - DermLite® handheld dermatoscope
> - FotoFinder® videodermatoscope
> - Folliscope®

Handyscope (FotoFinder Systems GmbH, Bad Birnbach, Germany) is a mobile-connected dermatoscope. The models for the iPhone 5S, 5, 6, and iPod Touch enable the taking of polarized and nonpolarized images. These models can also be used to take cross-polarized pictures without contact to the skin. The older models for iPhone 4, 4S, and 3GS only allow for polarized images. Handyscope allows for magnification up to 20×.

Veox DermScope (Canfield Imaging Systems, Fairfield, NJ, USA) is another mobile-connected dermatoscope for iPhone (4, 4S, and 5), iPod Touch, and iPad (2, 3, 4, and Air). It works in polarized and nonpolarized lighting modes and also allows for noncontact-polarized viewing. This device enables rotating of the dermatoscope lens out of the way for taking an overview photograph of the patient. The Veos DermScope takes images at a magnification of 10×. Its one-touch zoom allows for a magnification of 30×.

The DermLite handheld dermatoscope (3 Gen LLC, San Juan Capistrano, CA, USA) is a connecting kit for the iPhone 4, 4S, 5, 5S, and 6, for the iPad 3, Air, and Mini, and for the Samsung Galaxy phone. The pictures obtained allow for 10× magnification. The DermLite handheld dermatoscope can also be connected with a digital camera; in this way, images can be enlarged to a magnification of 30× through an optical zoom lens.

FotoFinder (FotoFinder Systems GmbH, Bad Birnbach, Germany) videodermatoscope is an immersion dermoscopy nonpolarized system with a videocamera equipped with lenses providing magnifications ranging from 20× to 70×. The images obtained are visualized on a monitor and stored on a personal computer. A polarization kit is available for polarized dermoscopy.

Folliscope (LeadM Corp, Seoul, South Korea) is an automated digital phototrichogram system. It is a simple USB connection-based device that is connected to a computer and screen. It can automatically measure different trichological parameters including hair density, hair shaft diameter, and the proportions of different hair types.

Quality of images varies depending on the instrument; videodermatoscopes usually provide the best images for nonpolarized dermoscopy. Magnification of iPhone-connected dermatoscopes varies depending on instruments: 20× for the Handyscope, 12.5× for the DermScope, and 10× for the DermLite.

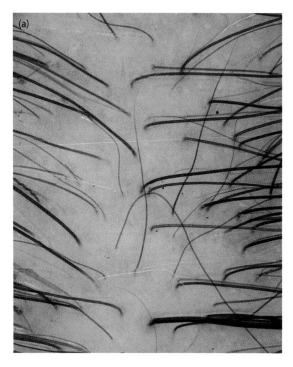

(a)

Figure 3.1 Images from the same scalp area taken with the FotoFinder videodermatoscope (a), the Handyscope (b), and the Veos DermScope (c). (*Continued*)

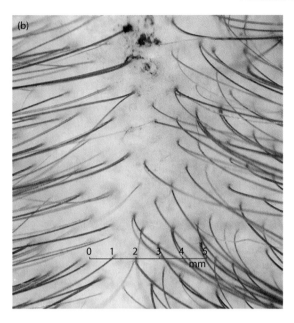
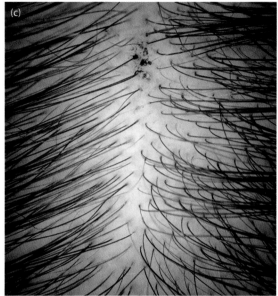

Figure 3.1 (Continued) Images from the same scalp area taken with the FotoFinder videodermatoscope (a), the Handyscope (b), and the Veos DermScope (c).

HOW TO EXAMINE THE SCALP

Box 3.2 How to Examine the Scalp (Figures 3.2 through 3.6)

- Diffuse/patterned alopecias: Vertex, mid, and frontal scalp after central parting and occipital scalp as control.
- Patchy alopecias: Center and periphery of the patch. Use polarized dermoscopy for scales and peripilar casts.
- Marginal alopecias: Evaluate the hairline to assess the presence/absence of vellus hairs. Use polarized dermoscopy for scales and peripilar casts.
- Inherited hair shaft disorders: Evaluate the occipital scalp, eyebrows, and eyelashes.
- Acquired hair shaft disorders: Examine the distal shaft and the hair fragments obtained with the pull/tug test. Polarized dermoscopy provides better images.

Scalp examination depends on the type of hair loss: diffuse versus patchy and nonscarring versus scarring. In general, polarized dermoscopy allows for better visualization of scales and is preferred for all types of scarring alopecia. Epiluminescence nonpolarized dermoscopy provides better visualization of vascular patterns.

In diffuse and patterned alopecia, it is important to part the hair in the midline and examine three areas on the top of the scalp (vertex, mid scalp, and frontal 2–3 cm from the hairline). The occipital region should also be examined as a control area, usually the mid occipital and lower occipital. For nonpolarized dermoscopy, alcohol or spring thermal water can be used as a liquid medium. It is always important to clean the lens with alcohol before each patient. I usually take a 20× and 50× image from each area. Further images are taken when a particular feature is seen.

In patchy alopecia, examine the center of the patch first to establish whether it is nonscarring (presence of follicular openings) or scarring (absence of follicular openings). In case of nonscarring alopecias, it is important to evaluate the apparently normal scalp in order to establish disease diffusion. In case of scarring alopecia, always perform a polarized examination of the periphery of the patch to look for peripilar casts or keratotic plugs.

(a)
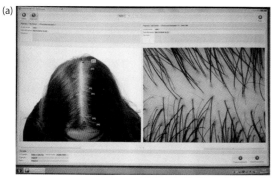

(b)
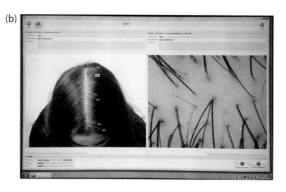

(c)
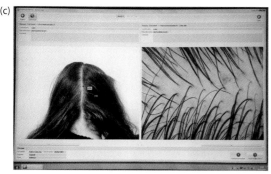

Figure 3.2 Scalp examination in a case of diffuse or patterned alopecia. Parting pictures are taken from the vertex, mid, and frontal scalp (a). At each site, pictures at high magnification (50×) are useful to assess variability (b). The occipital scalp is also evaluated as a control (c).

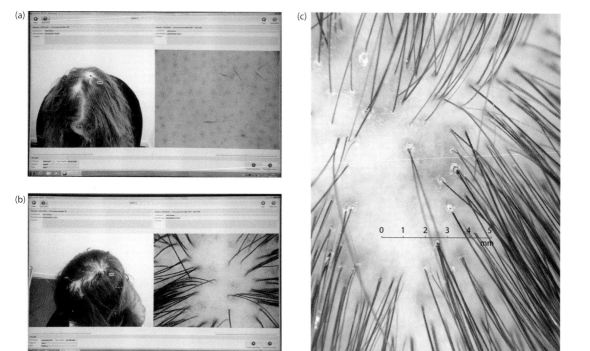

Figure 3.3 Scalp examination in a case of patchy alopecia. Yellow dots, corresponding to follicular openings, indicate nonscarring alopecia (a). The absence of follicular openings suggests scarring alopecia (b). Polarized dermoscopy is used to identify peripilar casts (c).

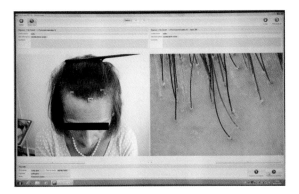

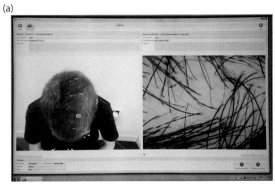

(a)

Figure 3.4 Scalp examination in a case of marginal alopecia. The absence of vellus hairs and peripilar casts suggests frontal fibrosing alopecia.

In marginal alopecia, always examine the hairline for the presence of vellus hairs, which are typically absent in frontal fibrosing alopecia. Use polarized dermoscopy to look for peripilar casts and hair casts.

In congenital hair shaft disorders, it is important to examine the whole scalp, starting from the occipital area, which is usually the site where the hair breakage is more evident. Always check the eyebrows and eyelashes, which may be the only site of involvement in older patients.

In acquired hair shaft disorders, it is important to look for signs of weathering, particularly trichorrhexis nodosa in the distal shaft. Always use the dermatoscope, and it is better to use polarized dermoscopy to evaluate signs of breakage in the hair fragments obtained with the pull/tug test.

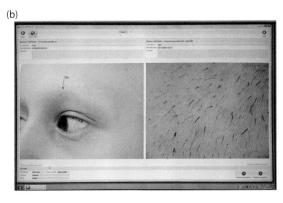

(b)

Figure 3.5 Scalp examination in a patient with monilethrix. Examination of the scalp (a) and eyebrows (b).

SUGGESTED READINGS

Arrazola P, Mullani NA, Abramovits W. DermLite II: An innovative por instrument for dermoscopy without the need of immersion fluids. *Skinmed.* 2005 Mar–Apr; 4(2):78–83.

Karadağ Köse Ö, Güleç AT. Clinical evaluation of alopecias using a handheld dermatoscope. *J Am Acad Dermatol.* 2012 Aug;67(2):206–14.

Nikam VV, Mehta HH. A nonrandomized study of trichoscopy patterns using non polarized (contact) and polarized (noncontact) dermatoscopy in hair and shaft disorders. *Int J Trichol.* 2014 Apr;6(2):54–62.

Rogers NE. Scoping scalp disorders: Practical use of a novel dermatoscope to diagnose hair and scalp conditions. *J Drugs Dermatol.* 2013 Mar;12(3):283–90.

Silverberg NB, Silverberg JI, Wong ML. Trichoscopy using a handheld dermoscope: An in-office technique to diagnose genetic disease of the hair. *Arch Dermatol.* 2009 May;145(5):600–1.

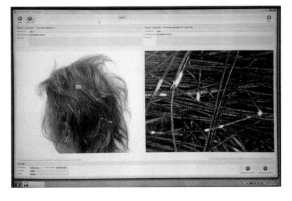

Figure 3.6 Examination of the hair shafts in a patient with cosmetic weathering.

4 Nonscarring alopecias
Colombina Vincenzi and Antonella Tosti

MALE PATTERN HAIR LOSS/ ANDROGENETIC ALOPECIA

> *Box 4.1* Male Pattern Hair Loss (Figures 4.1 through 4.7)
>
> - Most common form of hair loss in men
> - Progressive reduction in the diameter, length, and pigmentation of the hair
> - Hair thinning limited to androgen-dependent scalp regions
> - Dermoscopy: Hair diameter diversity, peripilar signs, and yellow dots

Male pattern hair loss (MPHL) affects up to 80% of men in the course of their life and is caused by a progressive reduction in the diameter, length, and pigmentation of the hair. Hair thinning is limited to the frontal, temporal, and vertex areas (androgen-dependent scalp regions) and results from the effects of the testosterone metabolite dihydrotestosterone (DHT) on androgen-sensitive hair follicles. Androgen sensitivity is genetically determined and depends on DHT production through 5-alpha reductase enzymes.

MPHL involves the fronto-temporal areas and the vertex, following a pattern that corresponds to the Hamilton–Norwood scale.

MPHL is a progressive disease that tends to worsen with time.

Medical treatments of MPHL include 5% topical minoxidil and/or the oral type II 5-alpha reductase inhibitor finasteride 1 mg. Treatment should be prolonged over time to maintain efficacy.

Dermoscopic features
Hair diameter diversity: The presence of hairs with different calibers is typical of androgenetic alopecia and reflects progressive hair miniaturization due to the disease. This has also been described with the term "anisotrichosis" and is better assessed using high magnification (50×).

A diversity of >20% is diagnostic of androgenetic alopecia.

Dermoscopy is very useful for detecting early androgenetic alopecia and for differential diagnosis with telogen effluvium. Severity of androgenetic alopecia can be evaluated using a photographic scale that considers hair diameter and density.

Short vellus hairs: These are a sign of severe miniaturization. They are more numerous on the vertex and temporal areas.

Peripilar sign: This sign is characterized by the presence of a brown depressed halo of approximately 1 mm in diameter at the follicular ostium around the emergent hair shaft. The peripilar sign is most commonly found in subjects with a high hair density score and is linked to perifollicular inflammation. We still do not know the prognostic significance of this sign, which is commonly found in patients with early androgenetic alopecia.

Yellow dots: These are a sign of severe miniaturization and are numerous in patients with severe baldness. They correspond to follicular ostia filled with keratin and sebum.

Pinpoint white dots: The sun-exposed scalp of patients with severe MPHL shows pinpoint white dots, which correspond to empty follicular ostia and sweat gland openings.

Scalp pigmentation: This is commonly observed on the scalps of patients with androgenetic alopecia as a consequence of sun exposure. Pigmentation has a typical honeycomb-like pattern.

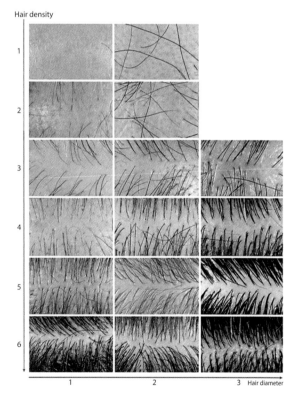

Figure 4.1 Photographic scale for evaluating severity using diameter and density. (From de Lacharrière O, et al. *Arch Dermatol.* 2001 May;137(5):641–6. With permission.)

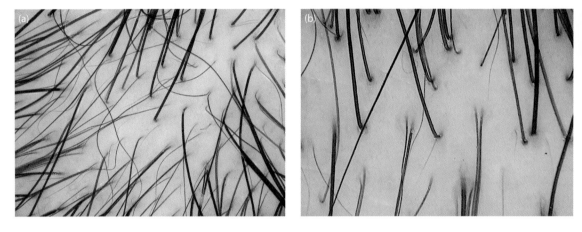

Figure 4.2 (a, b) Hair diameter diversity: there is variability in hair thickness with hair shafts of different thicknesses and lengths.

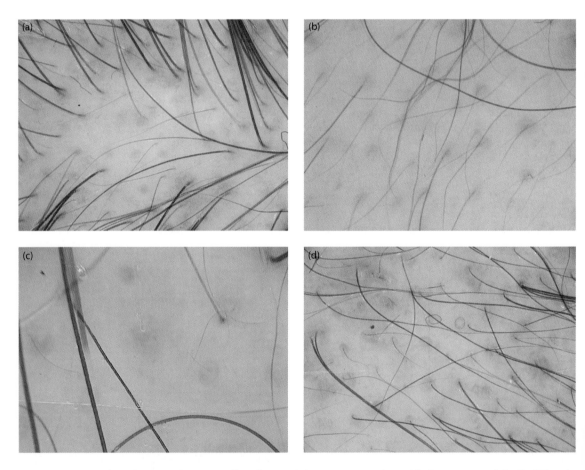

Figure 4.3 MPHL: hair diameter diversity, yellow dots, and short regrowing hairs (a); dermoscopy of the "bald" scalp shows yellow dots and short regrowing hairs but minimal variability, as most hairs are already miniaturized (b); and yellow dots at high magnification in which some are empty and others contain short vellus hairs (c); note numerous short vellus hairs and circle hairs (d).

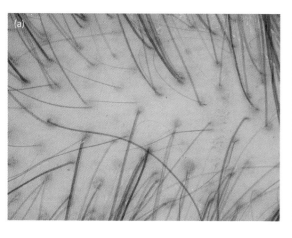
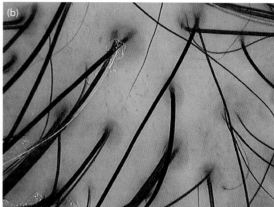

Figure 4.4 (a, b) Peripilar sign: the emergent hair shaft is surrounded by a brown depressed halo.

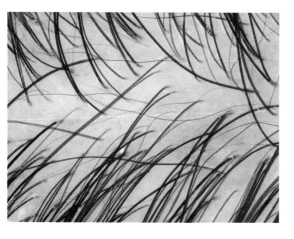

Figure 4.5 MPHL hair diameter diversity and honeycomb pattern due to sun exposure.

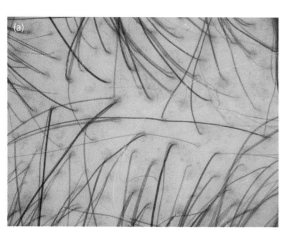
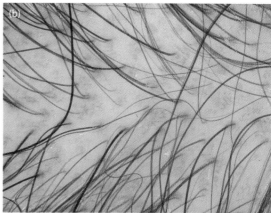

Figure 4.6 MPHL: dermoscopy enables the observation of improvement after treatment: before (a) and after (b) treatment with finasteride 1 mg for 6 months.

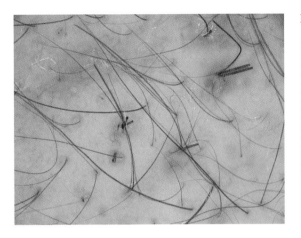

Figure 4.7 MPHL after hair transplantation. Dermoscopy shows hair regrowth.

FEMALE PATTERN HAIR LOSS

Box 4.2 Female Pattern Hair Loss (Figures 4.8 through 4.11)

- Affects up to 50% of women
- Progressive reduction in the diameter, length, and pigmentation of the hair
- Hair thinning limited to androgen-dependent scalp regions or diffuse
- Dermoscopy: Hair diameter diversity, peripilar signs, yellow dots, and short vellus hair on the frontal scalp

Female pattern hair loss (FPHL) affects up to 50% of women in their lifetime and produces diffuse thinning of the crown region with maintenance of the frontal hairline (Ludwig pattern). Making a central parting and comparing hair density at the top with hair density at the occipital region can easily demonstrate this.

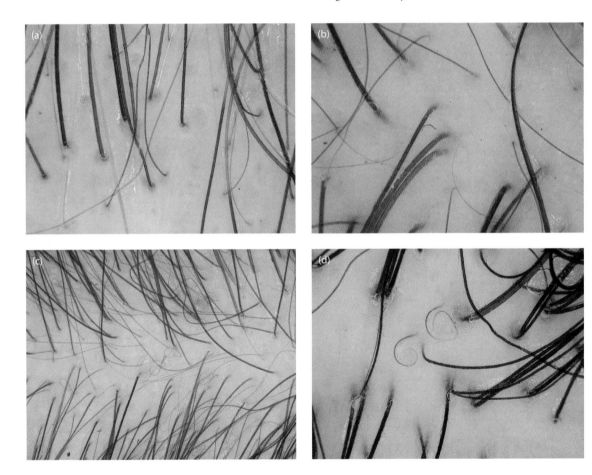

Figure 4.8 FPHL: hair shaft variability and yellow dots (a); hair shaft variability; most follicular units consist of a single hair (b); hair shaft variability, short regrowing hairs, and coiled hairs (c, d).

In premenopausal women, FPHL can be a sign of hyperandrogenism, together with hirsutism and acnes.

The dermoscopic features are similar to those described for MPHL and include:

Hair diameter diversity: A diversity of >20% is diagnostic for androgenetic alopecia. Dermoscopy is very useful for distinguishing FPHL from acute and chronic telogen effluvium. In women with severe FPHL, most follicular units consist of a single hair shaft.

Short vellus hairs (<0.03 mm): These are a sign of severe miniaturization. Their presence in the frontal scalp is a very useful clue for diagnosis. FPHL can be diagnosed when 10% or more than seven vellus hairs are detected in the frontal scalp.

Peripilar sign: This sign is commonly found in patients with early FPHL.

Yellow dots: These are a sign of severe miniaturization and are more numerous in patients with severe FPHL. More than four yellow dots in four images from the frontal scalp at high magnification (70×) are considered a major criterion for diagnosis.

Pinpoint white dots: The sun-exposed scalp can reveal this feature in very severe cases.

Scalp pigmentation: A honeycomb-like pattern is seen in sun-exposed areas.

Focal atrichia: Postmenopausal women often present with small bald areas, which at dermoscopy show follicular openings and very thin and short vellus hairs.

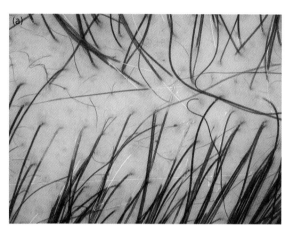
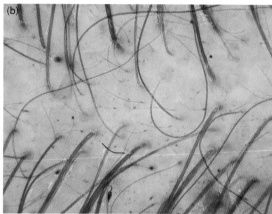

Figure 4.9 FPHL: short vellus hairs in the frontal scalp (a). Note the residues of hair dye on the scalp and within the follicular ostia (b).

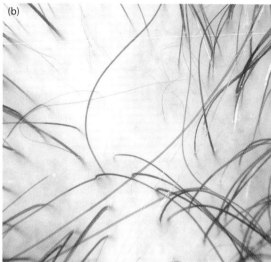
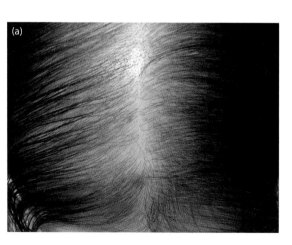

Figure 4.10 FPHL: focal atrichia: the patient presents with small alopecic patches (a) that show short vellus hairs at dermoscopy (b).

(a)

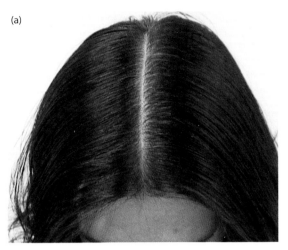

(b)

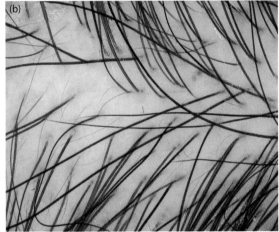

Figure 4.11 Early androgenetic alopecia in a young woman. Clinical examination reveals minimal thinning (a), but dermoscopy reveals hair diameter diversity (b).

ALOPECIA AREATA

> *Box 4.3* Alopecia Areata (Figures 4.12 through 4.23)
>
> - Nonscarring hair loss affecting 1%–2% of the general population.
> - T cell-mediated autoimmune disease affecting genetically predisposed individuals.
> - Single/multiple patches of hair loss that may progress to affect the whole scalp or all body hairs.
> - Dermoscopy: Yellow dots, exclamation mark hairs, dystrophic hairs, black dots, flame hairs, short regrowing hairs, circle hairs, caudability, and pseudo-monilethrix.
> - Dermoscopy is useful to establish disease activity and assess responses to treatment.

Alopecia areata is a common nonscarring alopecia characterized by acute patchy hair loss without scalp inflammation.

The disease may occur at any age and frequently affects children. A family history is present in approximately 30% of patients.

Alopecia areata most commonly affects the scalp, but it may involve the beard, eyelashes, eyebrows and pubic, axillary and body hair.

Diagnosis of alopecia areata is quite simple in typical cases. Disease activity can be evaluated by the pull test and by the presence of dystrophic and exclamation mark hairs upon scalp examination.

Dermoscopic features
Yellow dots

Yellow dots are a characteristic finding of alopecia areata in Caucasians and Asians. They appear as round or polycyclic yellow to yellow–pink dots, which may be devoid of hair or contain miniaturized short regrowing hairs, black dots, exclamation mark hairs, or broken hairs. Yellow dots correspond to keratin- and sebum-filled infundibula and are not visible in children before puberty. They are not seen in the black scalp.

White dots

Pigmented scalps show pinpoint white dots instead of yellow dots. These may be empty or contain vellus hairs, broken hairs, or black dots.

Broken hairs

Dermoscopy clearly shows all degrees of broken hair shafts with fractured tips. Broken hairs are not exclusive to alopecia areata, as they are also seen in trichotillomania and in chemotherapy alopecia. Exclamation mark hairs are characteristic of alopecia areata and appear as broken hairs with a thickened, pigmented tip. In acute alopecia areata, dystrophic and exclamation mark hairs are numerous.

Black dots

Black dots correspond to shafts that have fractured before emergence from the scalp (cadaverized hairs). Although a few black dots are seen in numerous conditions in addition to scarring alopecias, the presence of numerous black dots is highly suggestive of alopecia areata.

Flame hairs

These are wavy and cone-shaped hair residues with a flame appearance; they are usually seen in acute disease and pathologically correspond to pigmented casts.

Caudability

This dermoscopic feature describes proximal narrowing of the hair shaft and is typically seen at the periphery of enlarging patches.

Pseudo-monilethrix: The hair shaft may present multiple restrictions, and this finding is limited to a few hairs.

Short regrowing miniaturized hairs/circle hairs

This is a common feature seen in both acute and chronic alopecia areata. They represent the miniaturized nanogen hairs. In some cases, they are coiled (circle hairs). The presence of numerous circle hairs is very suggestive of a diagnosis of alopecia areata.

Dermoscopy is useful for evaluating disease activity and responses to treatment.

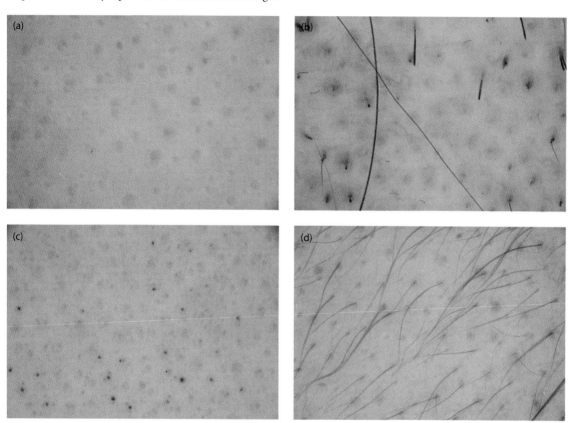

Figure 4.12 Alopecia areata. Yellow dots: the yellow dots can be empty (a) or contain broken hairs (b), black dots (c), or vellus-like hairs (d).

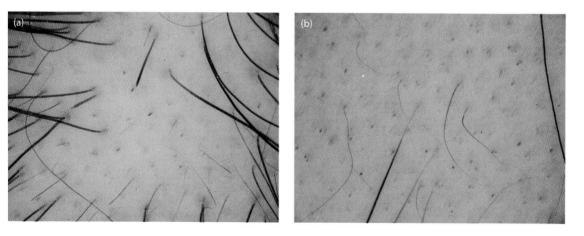

Figure 4.13 Alopecia areata in children. The follicular openings are of the same color as the scalp and contain broken hairs, exclamation mark hairs (a), black dots (b), or vellus and circle hairs (c).   (*Continued*)

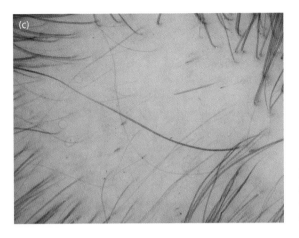

Figure 4.13 (*Continued*) Alopecia areata in children. The follicular openings are of the same color as the scalp and contain broken hairs, exclamation mark hairs (a), black dots (b), or vellus and circle hairs (c).

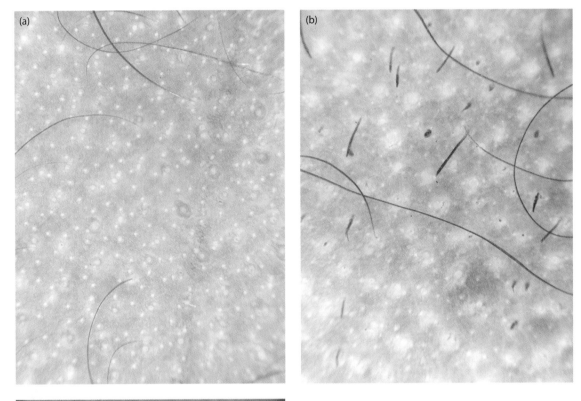

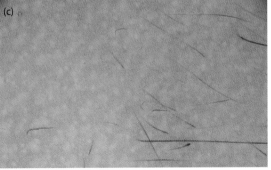

Figure 4.14 Alopecia areata in the pigmented scalp. Pinpoint white dots: as with yellow dots, the pinpoint white dots can be empty (a) or contain broken hairs and exclamation mark hairs or black dots (b). The sun-exposed scalp of Caucasians also shows pinpoint white dots instead of yellow dots (c).

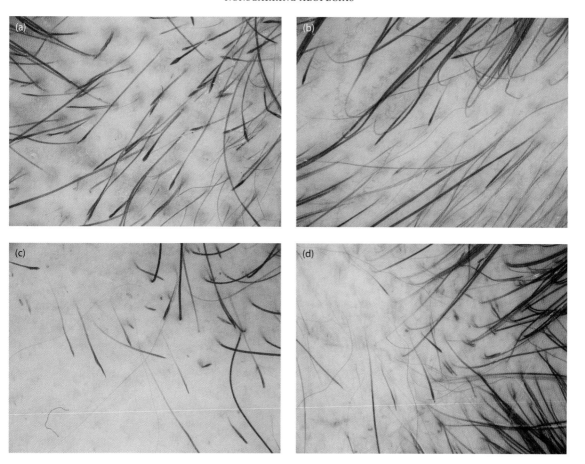

Figure 4.15 Alopecia areata. Exclamation mark hairs: the broken shaft has a thick, darker, frayed tip (a, b, c). Vellus hairs can also show this sign (d).

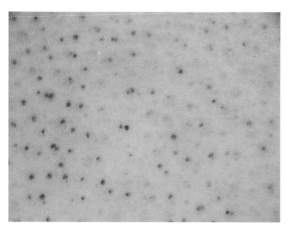

Figure 4.16 Alopecia areata. Black dots are a sign of acute disease.

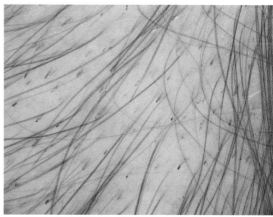

Figure 4.17 Alopecia areata. Flame hairs: these are usually interspersed with black dots.

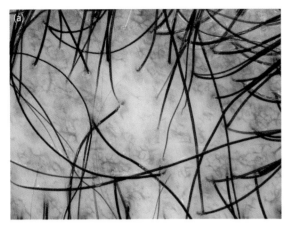
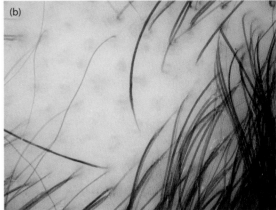

Figure 4.18 Alopecia areata. Caudability (a, b).

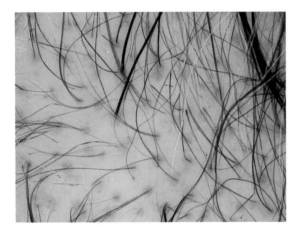

Figure 4.19 Alopecia areata. Pseudo-monilethrix.

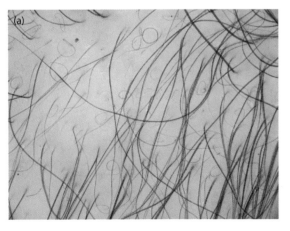
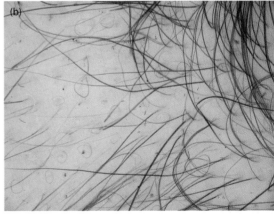

Figure 4.20 Alopecia areata. Circle hairs: the presence of numerous circle hairs is very suggestive of a diagnosis of alopecia areata. Circle hairs may be the only feature (a) or may be associated broken hairs (b) or with black dots and flame hairs in very acute disease (c). *(Continued)*

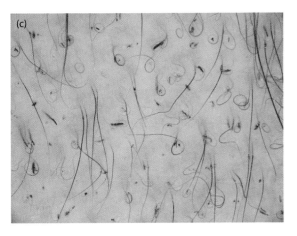

Figure 4.20 (Continued) Alopecia areata. Circle hairs: the presence of numerous circle hairs is very suggestive of a diagnosis of alopecia areata. Circle hairs may be the only feature (a) or may be associated broken hairs (b) or with black dots and flame hairs in very acute disease (c).

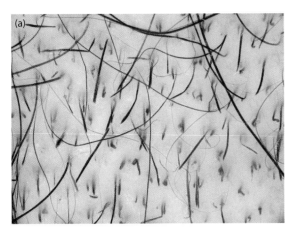

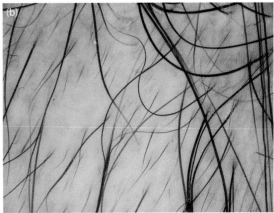

Figure 4.21 Dermoscopy in the follow-up of alopecia areata. Acute relapse with exclamation mark and flame hairs (a) versus diffuse hair regrowth (b).

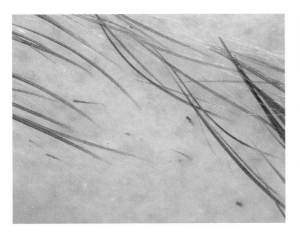

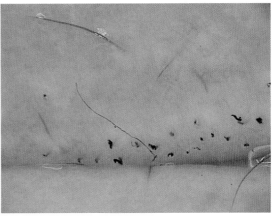

Figure 4.22 Alopecia areata of the eyebrows: dermoscopy shows dystrophic and exclamation mark hairs.

Figure 4.23 Alopecia areata of the eyelashes: dermoscopy shows flame hairs.

ALOPECIA AREATA INCOGNITO

Box 4.4 Alopecia Areata Incognito (Figures 4.24 and 4.25)

- Diffuse hair thinning without typical patches of alopecia.
- Usually affects women, and thinning may be more evident on androgen-dependent scalp.
- Positive pull test: Microscopy shows telogen hairs.
- Dermoscopy: Yellow dots and short miniaturized regrowing hairs.

Alopecia areata incognito, first described by Rebora in 1987, is a variety of alopecia areata characterized by diffuse hair shedding in the absence of typical patches. The prevalence of alopecia areata incognito is unknown and its diagnosis requires a scalp biopsy.

In our experience, these patients are often misdiagnosed as having telogen effluvium, diffuse alopecia, or androgenetic alopecia.

The disease usually affects women who complain of acute diffuse hair thinning, which is often more severe on the androgen-dependent areas of the scalp.

Dermoscopy shows the presence of numerous yellow dots and short regrowing tip-shaped miniaturized hairs (2–4 mm long). The pattern is easily seen at all magnifications.

The diagnosis is confirmed by histopathology showing a preserved number of follicular units with decreased numbers of terminal follicles and a decreased terminal: vellus ratio, dilated infundibula, and the presence of "follicles of indeterminate stage of the cycle" observed at the level of lower and mid follicles.

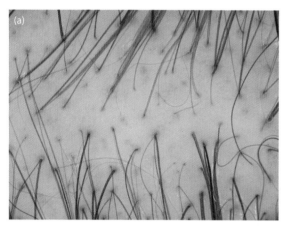
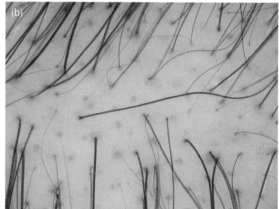
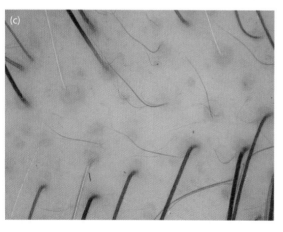

Figure 4.24 (a, b, c) Dermoscopy shows yellow dots and miniaturized regrowing hairs, as well as hair shaft variability.

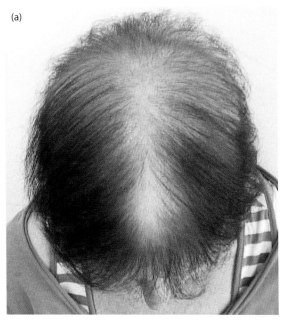

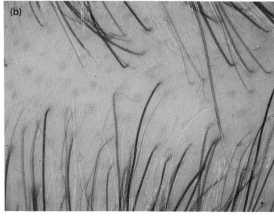

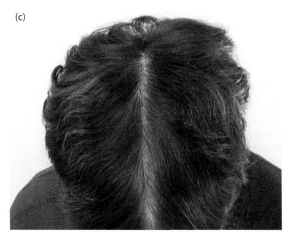

Figure 4.25 Alopecia areata incognito: severe diffuse thinning (a) and dermoscopy shows variability, yellow dots, and short regrowing hairs (b). Complete hair regrowth is shown after treatment with clobetasol propionate under occlusion (c).

ACUTE TELOGEN EFFLUVIUM

Box 4.5 Acute Telogen Effluvium (Figures 4.26 and 4.27)

- Acute hair shedding with/without visible thinning.
- The triggering factor is usually identified 2–4 months before onset.
- Positive pull test: Microscopy shows telogen hairs.
- Dermoscopy: Short regrowing hairs that may show variability.

Patients with acute telogen effluvium complain of severe hair shedding. Hair density can be normal or reduced, depending on the severity of the shedding and associated diseases. Acute telogen effluvium, in fact, often precipitates the onset of androgenetic alopecia or complicates the course of this condition.

History usually enables a tracing of the triggering factor 2–4 months before disease onset. The most common causes include medications, systemic illness, delivery, weight loss, nutritional deficiencies, and inflammatory scalp disorders. The pull test is positive with the extraction of telogen hairs.

Dermoscopy is not useful for diagnosis as it does not show any specific features. Short regrowing hairs are usually evident and it is important to reassure the patient. Hair shaft variability is observed in patients with associated androgenetic alopecia.

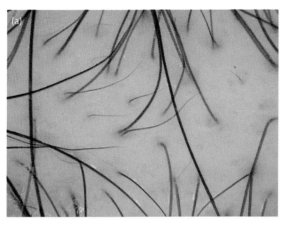
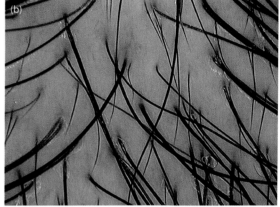

Figure 4.26 (a, b) Acute telogen effluvium. Short regrowing hair of normal thickness.

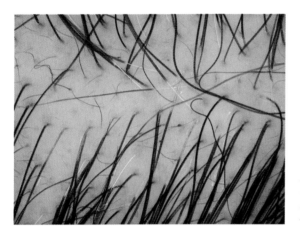

Figure 4.27 Acute telogen effluvium in a patient with androgenetic alopecia: note the short regrowing hairs of normal thickness, short vellus hairs, and hair shaft variability.

CHRONIC TELOGEN EFFLUVIUM

Box 4.6 Chronic Telogen Effluvium (Figure 4.28)

- Patient complains of hair shedding and bitemporal thinning.
- Hair mass looks normal, although it is considerably reduced according to the patient.
- Negative pull test: Microscopy shows telogen hairs.
- Dermoscopy: Absence of variability and short regrowing hairs.

Chronic telogen effluvium most commonly affects middle-aged women. Patients complain of increased shedding (often bringing bags of hairs to prove this), reduction of the hair mass, and bitemporal thinning. Clinical examination shows a normal density and the pull test is usually negative.

Dermoscopy shows an absence of variability and, in some cases, short regrowing hairs of normal thickness.

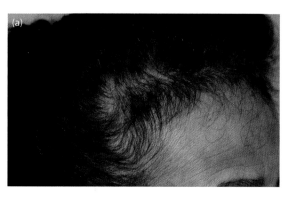
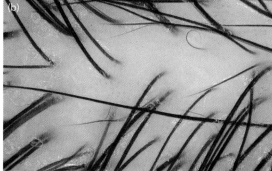

Figure 4.28 Normal density with bi-temporal recession (a). Short regrowing hairs of normal thickness and no hair shaft variability (b).

TRICHOTILLOMANIA

Box 4.7 Trichotillomania (Figures 4.29 through 4.32)

- Chronic compulsive disorder most commonly seen in children.
- Single/multiple irregular alopecia patches on the scalp; it may affect the eyebrows and/or eyelashes.
- Alopecic patches are covered with broken hairs of different lengths.
- Dermoscopy: Broken hairs, black dots, question mark hairs, longitudinally split short hairs, flame hairs, and hair powder.

Trichotillomania is a compulsive disorder characterized by an irresistible impulse of hair pulling. It is a relatively common cause of alopecia in children.

Hair pulling most commonly involves the scalp with irregular patches of hair loss that often show bizarre borders. Over the long term, the disorder may lead to scarring alopecia.

The affected areas are not completely bald but show short broken hairs of different lengths. Patients often deny the habit and it may be difficult to convince the parents of affected children of the diagnosis.

Dermoscopy is useful for showing evidence of pulling. The scalp shows broken hairs with a coiled tip (question mark hairs), broken hair shafts of various lengths that often show longitudinal splitting (hamburger sign), black dots, flame hairs, and hair dust. Yellow dots are often present. The main differential diagnosis of trichotillomania is alopecia areata, as broken hairs and flame hairs are seen in both conditions. Exclamation mark hairs, however, are not seen in trichotillomania. It is important to keep in mind that the two conditions may occur together.

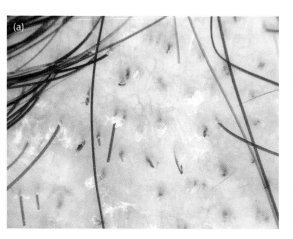
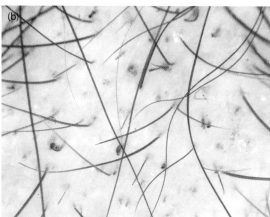

Figure 4.29 Trichotillomania: question mark hairs, broken hairs of different lengths, flame hairs, and black dots (a), several broken hairs show longitudinal splitting (b), and yellow dots are also evident (c). (*Continued*)

43

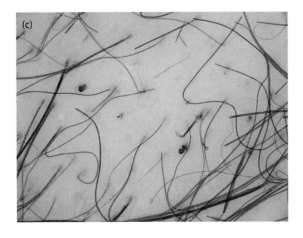

Figure 4.29 (Continued) Trichotillomania: question mark hairs, broken hairs of different lengths, flame hairs, and black dots (a), several broken hairs show longitudinal splitting (b), and yellow dots are also evident (c).

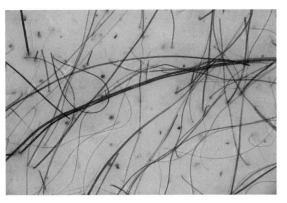

Figure 4.30 Trichotillomania: black dots and broken hairs; differential diagnosis with alopecia areata is impossible from this picture.

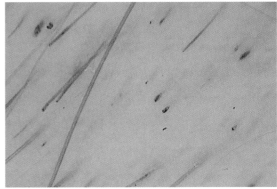

Figure 4.31 Trichotillomania: hair dust.

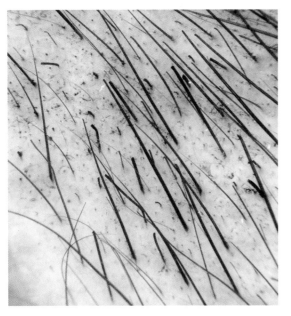

Figure 4.32 Trichotillomania of the eyebrows showing broken hairs and question mark hairs.

DISSECTING CELLULITIS

Box 4.8 Dissecting Cellulitis (Figures 4.33 through 4.36)

- Follicular occlusion disorder most commonly affecting black men.
- Multifocal painful nodules with sinus tracts discharging purulent material.
- Alopecia is reversible in early stages of the disease, but can become scarring in longstanding lesions.
- Dermoscopy: Yellow dots, black dots, and keratotic plugs.

Dissecting cellulitis of the scalp is a follicular occlusion disorder that may progressively lead to scarring alopecia. It presents with multifocal painful nodules and boggy plaques with alopecia, which is reversible in early-stage disease, but can become scarring in longstanding lesions. Keloid formation is typical.

Dermoscopy of the alopecic areas shows features of noncicatricial alopecias with yellow dots, black dots, and short regrowing hairs. Scalp inflammation with erythema, arborizing vessels, and giant capillaries is common. It is also typical to see large follicular openings filled with a keratotic plug.

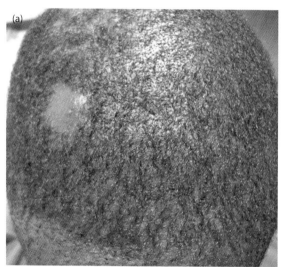

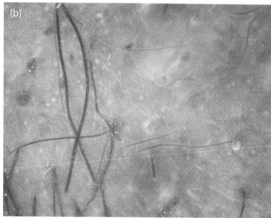

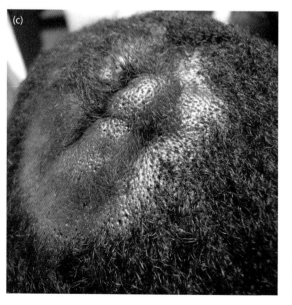

Figure 4.33 Dissecting cellulitis: in early-stage disease, the alopecia is nonscarring (a) and dermoscopy shows yellow dots, broken hairs, and keratotic plugs (b). However, the disease becomes scarring with keloid formation if the disease is left untreated (c).

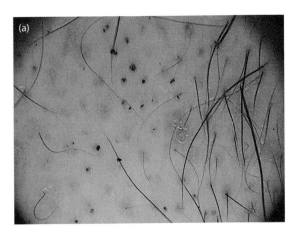
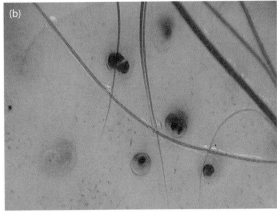

Figure 4.34 (a, b) Dissecting cellulitis: yellow dots, black dots, and short regrowing hairs.

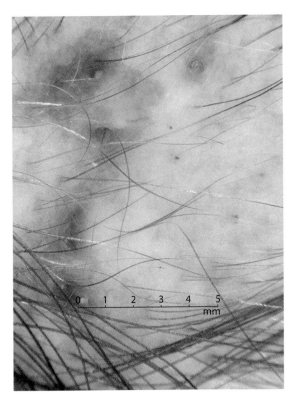
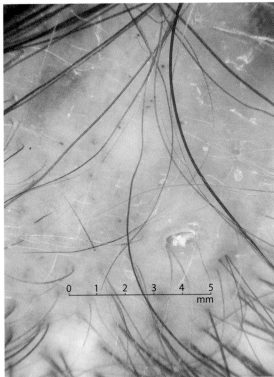

Figure 4.35 Dissecting cellulitis, inflammatory phase: scalp erythema, black dots, short regrowing hairs, and follicular plugging.

Figure 4.36 Dissecting cellulitis: black dots, broken hairs, and large keratotic plugs filling a prominent enlarged follicular opening.

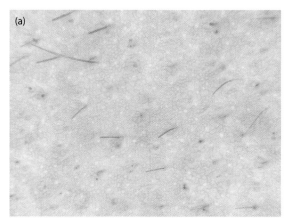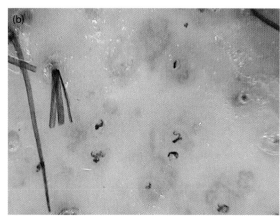

Figure 4.37 Chemotherapy alopecia: broken hairs, pinpoint white dots, and black dots in a patient of African descent (a); flame hairs (b).

CHEMOTHERAPY ALOPECIA

Box 4.9 Chemotherapy Alopecia (Figure 4.37)

- Severe anagen effluvium occurring during chemotherapy.
- The alopecia involves nearly all of the scalp hair, eyebrows, and eyelashes.
- Full regrowth is expected in the majority of cases, but permanent alopecia may occur with certain drugs.
- Dermoscopy: Yellow dots, black dots, flame hairs, acute constrictions, and color changes along the hair shaft, tapering hairs, and caudability hairs.

Chemotherapy alopecia is an acute and extreme form of anagen effluvium that is associated with antineoplastic agents. The hair loss begins within 7–10 days of drug administration and becomes more apparent with time. The alopecia involves nearly all of the scalp hair, eyebrows, and eyelashes. Patients usually prefer to shave their scalp to avoid the stress of seeing the severe shedding.

Dermoscopy shows findings that are very similar to those seen in alopecia areata, with yellow dots or pinpoint white dots in the black scalp, hair breakage, black dots, flame hairs, and caudability. Changes in the hair shaft color have also been reported.

RADIOTHERAPY ALOPECIA

Box 4.10 Radiotherapy Alopecia (Figures 4.38 and 4.39)

- Radiotherapy causes both anagen effluvium and cicatricial alopecia depending on dosages and durations.
- Single short-term exposure to 300–600 Gy of irradiation produces temporary epilation.
- Dermoscopy: Yellow dots, black dots, and flame hair.

Acute anagen effluvium due to radiotherapy can occur as a single patch of nonscarring alopecia or diffuse alopecia. This is seen after neurosurgical operations with fluoroscopic imaging. It can also occur in association with radiation alopecia in patients undergoing radiotherapy for brain tumors.

Dermoscopy shows features similar to alopecia areata, with yellow dots, black dots, and flame hairs.

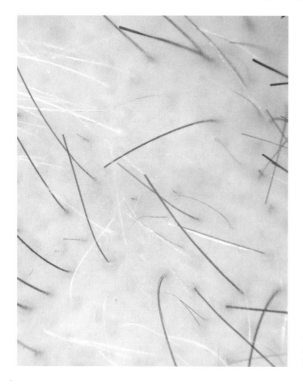

Figure 4.38 Anagen effluvium after radiation exposure during angioembolization: yellow dots, black dots, broken hairs, and short regrowing hairs.

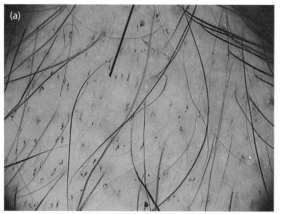

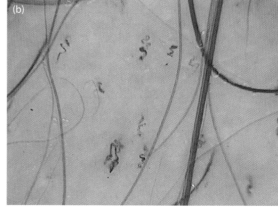

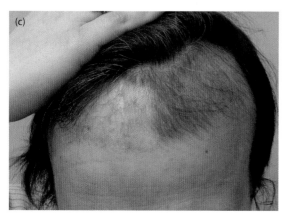

Figure 4.39 Flame hairs (a, b) in a patient undergoing radiotherapy for a brain tumor. Follow-up shows scarring alopecia of the area treated with high radiation dosages and hair regrowth on the scalp areas at the periphery of the field, which received low radiation dosages (c).

SUGGESTED READINGS

Ardigò M, Tosti A, Cameli N, Vincenzi C, Misciali C, Berardesca E. Reflectance confocal microscopy of the yellow dot pattern in alopecia areata. *Arch Dermatol.* 2011 Jan;147(1):61–4.

de Lacharrière O, Deloche C, Misciali C, Piraccini BM, Vincenzi C, Bastien P, Tardy I, Bernard BA, Tosti A. Hair diameter diversity: A clinical sign reflecting the follicle miniaturization. *Arch Dermatol.* 2001 May;137(5):641–6.

de Moura LH, Duque-Estrada B, Abraham LS, Barcaui CB, Sodre CT. Dermoscopy findings of alopecia areata in an African–American patient. *J Dermatol Case Rep.* 2008 Dec;2(4):52–4.

Herskovitz I, de Sousa IC, Tosti A. Vellus hairs in the frontal scalp in early female pattern hair loss. *Int J Trichol.* 2013 Jul;5(3):118–20.

Inui S, Nakajima T, Itami S. Scalp dermoscopy of androgenetic alopecia in Asian people. *J Dermatol.* 2009 Feb;36(2):82–5.

Inui S, Nakajima T, Itami S. Coudability hairs: A revisited sign of alopecia areata assessed by trichoscopy. *Clin Exp Dermatol.* 2010 Jun;35(4):361–5.

Inui S, Nakajima T, Nakagawa K, Itami S. Clinical significance of dermoscopy in alopecia areata: Analysis of 300 cases. *Int J Dermatol.* 2008 Jul;47(7):688–93.

Rakowska A, Slowinska M, Kowalska-Oledzka E, Olszewska M, Rudnicka L. Dermoscopy in female androgenic alopecia: Method standardization and diagnostic criteria. *Int J Trichol.* 2009 Jul;1(2):123–30.

Rakowska A, Slowinska M, Olszewska M, Rudnicka L. New trichoscopy findings in trichotillomania: Flame hairs, V-sign, hook hairs, hair powder, tulip hairs. *Acta Derm Venereol.* 2014 May;94(3):303–6.

Ross EK, Vincenzi C, Tosti A. Videodermoscopy in the evaluation of hair and scalp disorders. *J Am Acad Dermatol.* 2006 Nov;55(5):799–806.

Tosti A, Torres F, Miteva M. Dermoscopy of early dissecting cellulitis of the scalp simulates alopecia areata. *Actas Dermosifiliogr.* 2013 Jan;104(1):92–3.

Tosti A, Whiting D, Iorizzo M, Pazzaglia M, Misciali C, Vincenzi C, Micali G. The role of scalp dermoscopy in the diagnosis of alopecia areata incognita. *J Am Acad Dermatol.* 2008 Jul;59(1):64–7.

5 Primary scarring alopecias
Antonella Tosti

Primary scarring alopecias include several disorders that affect the hair follicle, destroy bulge stem cells, and cause permanent scarring. Dermoscopy is very useful for distinguishing these different diseases and is also useful for selecting the optimal biopsy site.

LICHEN PLANOPILARIS

Lichen planopilaris (LPP) is the most common cause of cicatricial alopecia. The disease most frequently affects middle-aged females. Scalp itching is usually severe and correlated with disease activity.

The scalp shows irregular areas of cicatricial alopecia and the follicles surrounding the alopecic areas show perifollicular erythema and papules.

In active disease, the pull test produces the painless extraction of anagen hair roots with thickened sheaths.

The disease usually has a slowly progressive course and may result in severe alopecia.

The most characteristic dermoscopic features include the absence of follicular openings and peripilar casts presenting as concentrically arranged layers of scales around the hair shaft emergency. The presence of a group of two or three hairs surrounded by peripilar casts should raise the suspicion of LPP. Sometimes, a cast surrounds a tuft of four to five hairs. Vellus hairs are usually absent. Other dermoscopic findings include white patches, scalp erythema, broken hairs, pili torti, and blue–gray dots arranged in a target pattern around the follicular ostia. Vellus hairs are reduced or absent. Pinpoint white dots are seen in dark-skinned patients.

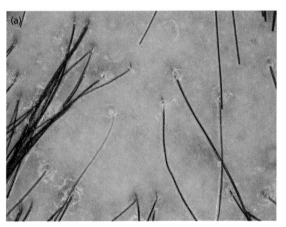
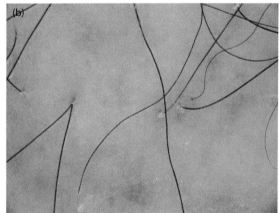

Figure 5.1 LPP: dermoscopy shows an absence of follicular openings and peripilar casts (a, b). In active disease, casts are thick and surround most of the emerging shafts (c). *(Continued)*

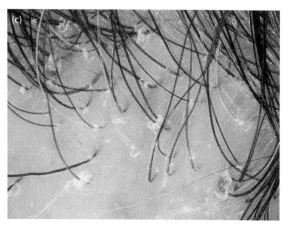

Figure 5.1 (Continued) LPP: dermoscopy shows an absence of follicular openings and peripilar casts (a, b). In active disease, casts are thick and surround most of the emerging shafts (c).

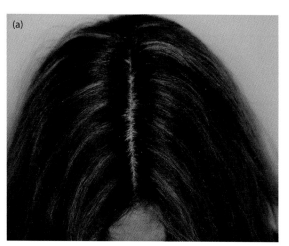

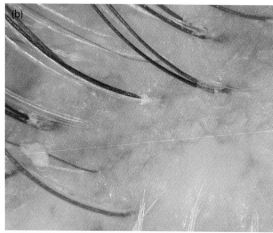

Figure 5.2 LPP: early disease presenting with scalp itching and few alopecic patches (a). Dermoscopy shows a loss of follicular openings and thin casts surrounding a group of two to three hair shafts emerging together (b).

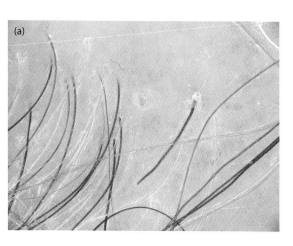

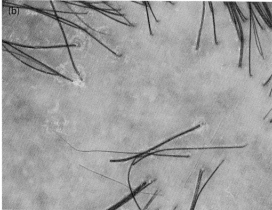

Figure 5.3 (a, b) LPP: broken hair shafts surrounded by peripilar casts are commonly observed.

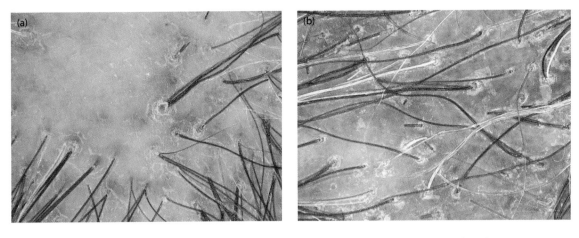

Figure 5.4 (a, b) LPP: very active disease with broken hair shafts, peripilar casts, and prominent erythema.

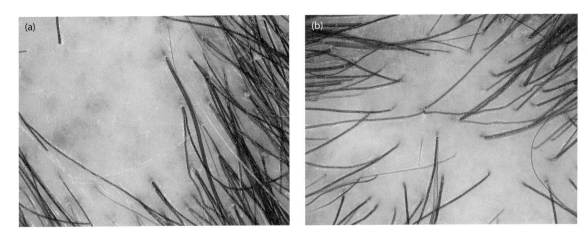

Figure 5.5 (a, b) LPP: pili torti are a frequent finding. Also note the absence of vellus hairs (a, b).

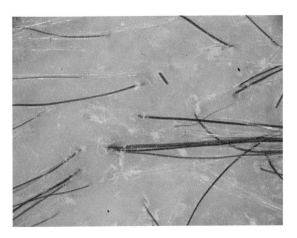

Figure 5.6 LPP: tuft of four hairs surrounded by a peripilar cast.

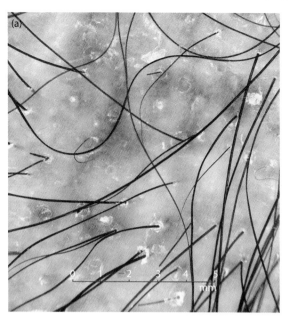

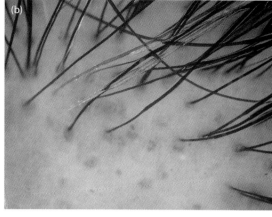

Figure 5.7 (a, b) LPP: blue–gray dots arranged in a target pattern around the follicular ostia.

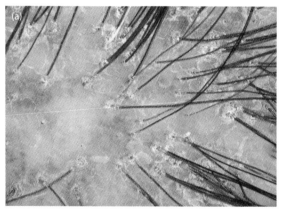

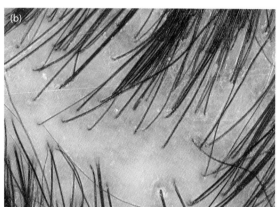

Figure 5.8 LPP: dermoscopy is useful for monitoring responses to treatment. In very active disease (a), the erythema and the peripilar casts are much improved after treatment with pioglitazone (b).

FRONTAL FIBROSING ALOPECIA

Box 5.3 Frontal Fibrosing Alopecia (Figures 5.9 through 5.18)

- Scarring alopecia causing progressive recession of the fronto-temporal hairline.
- Most commonly affects postmenopausal women.
- Band-like frontal alopecia with loss of follicular orifices, perifollicular erythema, and hyperkeratosis of the hair follicles at the hairline margin.
- Partial or complete loss of the eyebrows.
- Dermoscopy: Absence of vellus hair, peripilar casts, broken hairs, and black dots.

Frontal fibrosing alopecia is an uncommon variety of LPP that typically affects postmenopausal women. The patients complain of a slow, progressive recession of the fronto-temporal hairline. Partial or total alopecia of the eyebrows is frequently observed.

Clinical examination reveals a band of cicatricial alopecia in the fronto-temporal region; the cicatricial area is easily distinguished from the normal forehead by the absence of photoaging. The hair follicles at the hair margin show perifollicular erythema and hyperkeratosis.

Dermoscopy of the alopecic band reveals an absence of follicular openings. Dermoscopy of the hairline shows an absence of vellus hairs and peripilar casts surrounding the hair shafts at their emergence. Broken hairs and pili torti are commonly observed.

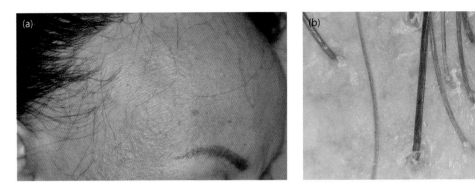

Figure 5.9 Frontal fibrosing alopecia: note the hairline recession, loss of the eyebrows and frontal papules (a). Dermoscopy shows the absence of vellus hairs and peripilar casts (b).

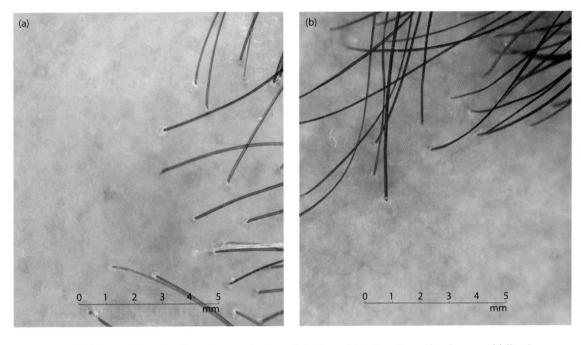

Figure 5.10 (a, b) Frontal fibrosing alopecia: examination of the frontal hairline shows the absence of follicular openings, the absence of vellus hairs, peripilar casts, and perifollicular erythema.

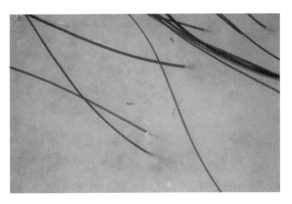

Figure 5.11 Frontal fibrosing alopecia: absence of vellus hairs, peripilar casts, and black dots.

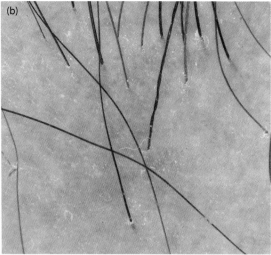

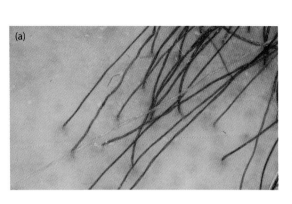

Figure 5.12 (a, b) Frontal fibrosing alopecia: absence of vellus hairs, peripilar casts, and pili torti.

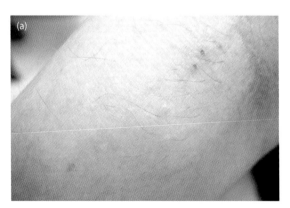

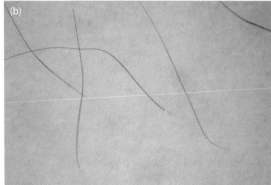

Figure 5.13 Frontal fibrosing alopecia: arm involvement (a). Dermoscopy shows peripilar casts (b).

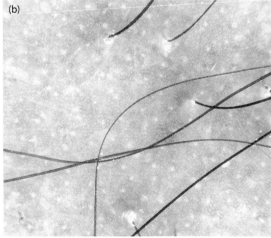

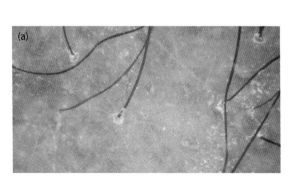

Figure 5.14 (a, b) Frontal fibrosing alopecia: the peripilar casts are usually thin, but in some cases can be more prominent.

Figure 5.15 Frontal fibrosing alopecia: the alopecic area shows irregular white patches of scarring.

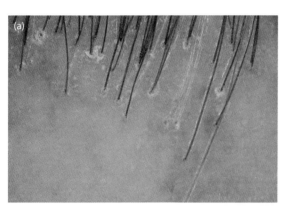
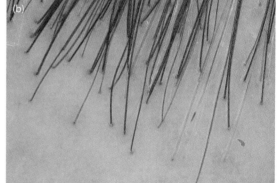

Figure 5.16 Frontal fibrosing alopecia before (a) and after treatment with an excimer laser (b). Note the reduction of the peripilar casts after therapy (b).

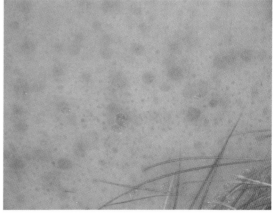

Figure 5.17 Frontal fibrosing alopecia: lichen planus pigmentosum is commonly associated with frontal fibrosing alopecia in patients with dark photo types. Dermoscopy shows granular gray–brown dots.

Figure 5.18 Frontal fibrosing alopecia: follicular red dots in the glabella.

DISCOID LUPUS ERYTHEMATOSUS

Box 5.4 Discoid Lupus Erythematosus (Figures 5.19 through 5.25)

- Cicatricial alopecia associated with active inflammatory lesions, atrophy, and telangiectasia.
- Scalp scaling is often a prominent feature.
- Loss of pigment is commonly seen in the black scalp.
- Dermoscopy: Loss of follicular openings, white patches, peripilar casts, keratotic plugs, red dots, enlarged branching vessels, and blue–gray dots in a speckled pattern in patients with dark skin.

Discoid lupus erythematosus (DLE) of the scalp is not common and may be associated with other cutaneous localizations of the disease.

Clinical examination reveals single or multiple alopecic patches. In active disease, the affected scalp is often edematous and shows erythema and scaling with follicular hyperkeratosis, atrophy and telangiectasia. Loss of pigment is typically seen in black patients. Diffuse and thick scales resembling scalp psoriasis are another possible presentation.

Tumid DLE may occasionally affect the scalp and produce alopecia. The disease usually presents in patches in which erythema and edema are prominent features. Scarring is not the rule.

Dermoscopy shows a loss of follicular openings as in all scarring alopecias. In some cases, the dermoscopic features resemble LPP with peripilar casts. Keratotic plugs are typical for DLE and can be a prominent feature in some patients. Red dots are erythematous polycyclic, concentric structures that correspond to dilated follicular openings surrounded by dilated vessels.

Their presence has been linked to early disease, and patches showing this pattern may regrow hair if promptly treated. Enlarged branching vessels are common and their presence strongly suggests diagnosis.

In patients with dark skin, blue–gray dots in a speckled pattern are commonly seen. These correspond to melanophages in the papillary dermis. The speckled pattern indicates that the incontinentia pigmenti is not limited to the follicles, but also affects the interfollicular epidermis.

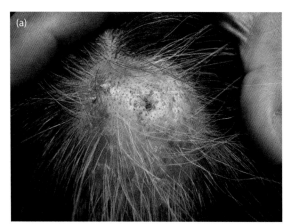

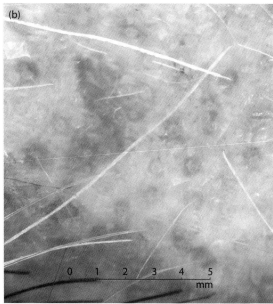

Figure 5.19 Edematous patch of alopecia with crust and scales (a). Dermoscopy shows a loss of follicular openings, loss of pigment, and keratotic plugs (b).

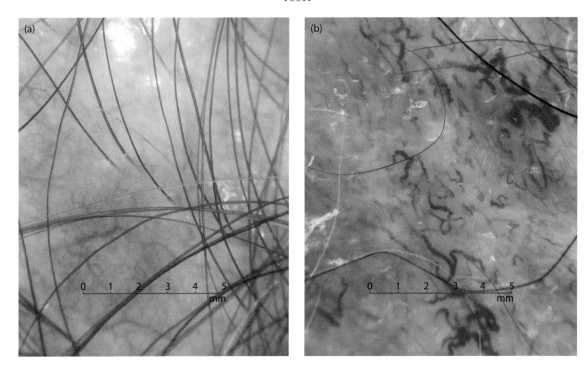

Figure 5.20 Enlarged branching vessels are very suggestive for diagnosis of DLE. The presence of giant capillaries indicates this diagnosis in this patient, who presented with peripilar casts (a), similar to LPP, together with enlarged branched vessels (b).

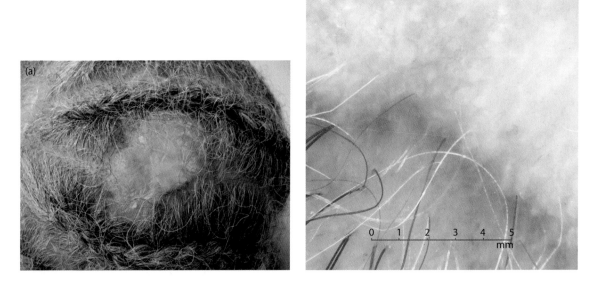

Figure 5.21 Loss of pigment is a typical feature in patients of color (a). Dermoscopy of the patch shows a loss of follicular openings, loss of pigment, and enlarged vessels (b).

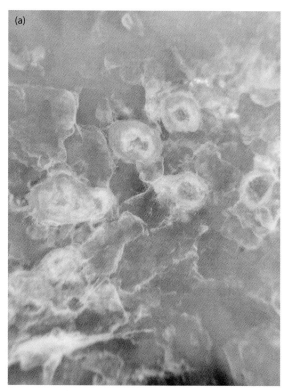

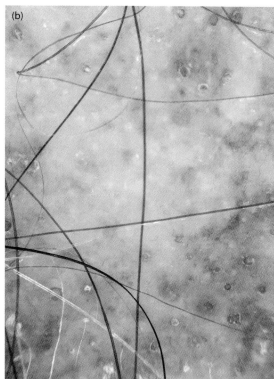

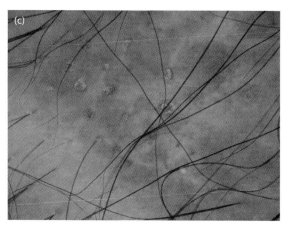

Figure 5.22 Keratotic plugs are also very typical (a). Loss of follicular openings, loss of pigment, and keratotic plugs are highly suggestive of this diagnosis (b). Keratotic plugs can be seen in association with peripilar casts (c).

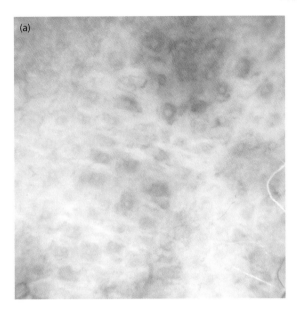

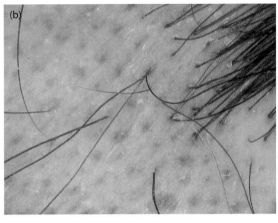

Figure 5.23 Red dots correspond to follicular openings surrounded by dilated vessels (a). Patches showing this pattern may regrow hair with treatment (b).

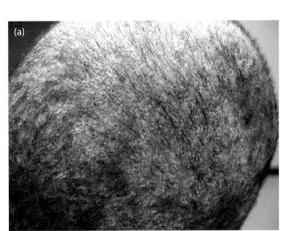

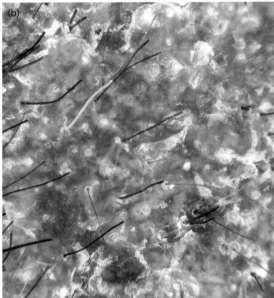

Figure 5.24 DLE presenting with diffuse thick scales and loss of pigment (a). Dermoscopy shows a loss of follicular openings, loss of pigment, and keratotic plugs (b).

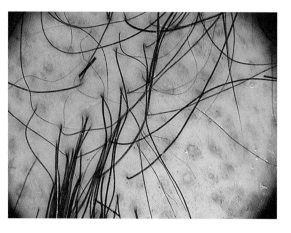

Figure 5.25 Blue–gray dots in a speckled pattern.

FOLLICULITIS DECALVANS

Box 5.5 Folliculitis Decalvans (Figures 5.26 through 5.31)

- Chronic scalp disorder characterized by severe recurrent scalp inflammation resulting in cicatricial alopecia.
- Papulo-pustular lesions, exudative crusted areas, cicatricial alopecia, and tufted folliculitis.
- Centrifugal progression is typical.
- Dermoscopy: Scalp edema with crusts and tufted hairs surrounded by thick concentric scales. Coiled dilated capillaries similar to those observed in scalp psoriasis. The presence of tufts of six or more hairs emerging together is highly suggestive of this diagnosis. Hair casts are commonly seen.

Folliculitis decalvans (FD) is a severe inflammatory scalp disorders that results in cicatricial alopecia with centrifugal progression. The scalp shows multiple recurrent papulo-pustular lesions and exudative crusted areas. The inflammation subsides when the follicles are destroyed.

Tufted folliculitis is typical and most commonly seen at the periphery of the patch. The disease may occasionally present with diffuse and thick scalp scales.

Dermoscopy shows severe scaling, pustular lesions and crusts. Peripilar casts are thicker than in LPP and surround the tufts of hairs. The presence of tufts of six or more hairs emerging together and surrounded by thick concentric scales is typical for FD. The presence of coiled capillary loops and hair tufting is also highly suggestive of this diagnosis. Hair casts are often seen around the proximal hair shafts, where they may surround a single shaft or several adjacent shafts. Sometimes, they can be seen in the middle and distal shafts.

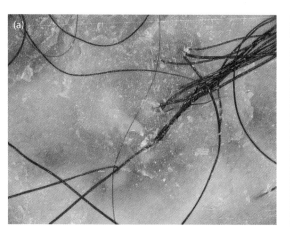
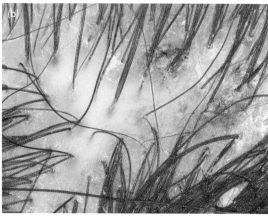

Figure 5.26 (a, b) FD: dermoscopy shows pustules as well as yellow and hemorrhagic crusts.

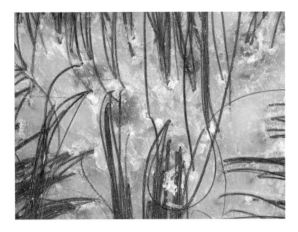

Figure 5.27 FD: severe scalp scaling with peripilar casts and yellow crusts.

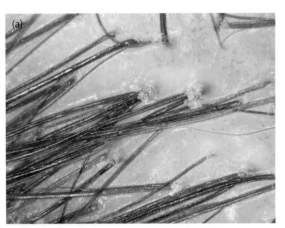

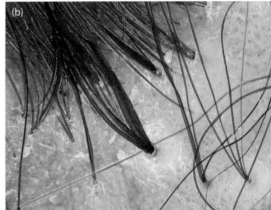

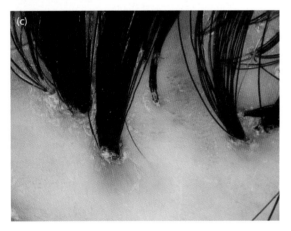

Figure 5.28 FD: presence of coiled vessels indicates this diagnosis even if tufts contain fewer than six hairs (a). Coiled vessels and the presence of tufts of more than six hairs (b, c).

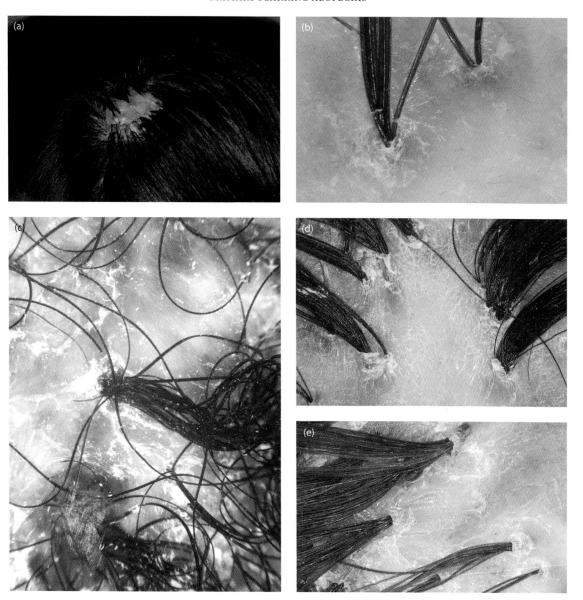

Figure 5.29 FD: patch of scarring alopecia with visible hair tufts at its periphery (a). Tufts of six hairs surrounded by thick concentric scales (b, c). Multiple tufts are commonly seen (d), with thick concentric scales surrounding the proximal hair shafts (e).

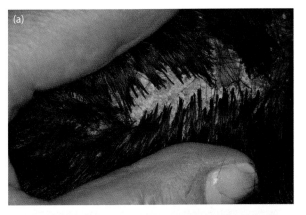

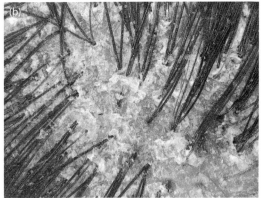

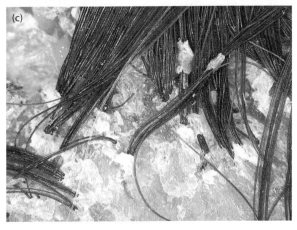

Figure 5.30 FD presenting with severe scalp scaling (a). Dermoscopy shows diffuse scaling with peripilar casts, hemorrhagic crusts (b) and hair tufts, which suggest this diagnosis (c). Also note the hair casts surrounding the proximal tufted shafts.

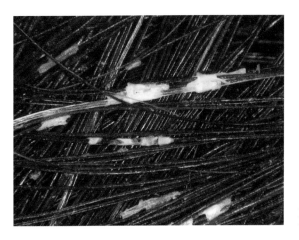

Figure 5.31 FD: hair casts can also be detected along the hair shaft's length.

ACNE KELOIDALIS NUCHAE

> *Box 5.6* Acne Keloidalis Nuchae (Figure 5.32)
>
> - Affects the occipital scalp and posterior neck and produces scarring alopecia.
> - Can be seen in association with dissecting cellulitis.
> - Relapsing painful papular and pustular lesions that produce hairless keloidal plaques.
> - Dermoscopy: Broken hairs, tufted hairs, and ingrown hairs.

Acne keloidalis nuchae is a chronic inflammatory condition that most commonly affects young men of African–American or Hispanic descent.

Shaving is considered a main factor for the development of the disease.

Dermoscopy shows broken hairs with tufting and peripilar casts.

CENTRAL CENTRIFUGAL CICATRICIAL ALOPECIA

> *Box 5.7* Central Centrifugal Cicatricial Alopecia (Figure 5.33)
>
> - Most common cause of scarring alopecia in women of African descent.
> - Alopecia of the central scalp that extends centrifugally.
> - Dermoscopy: Irregularly distributed pinpoint white dots and irregular white patches and peripilar white–gray halo surrounding the hairs within the patches.

Central centrifugal cicatricial alopecia (CCCA) is the most common cause of scarring alopecia among women of African descent. The disease presents with progressive

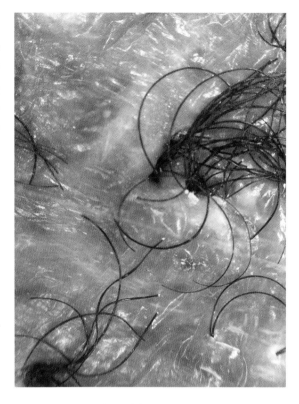

Figure 5.32 Acne keloidalis nuchae: dermoscopy shows tufting, scars, and pseudo-folliculitis with extrafollicular penetration.

central scalp hair loss, which starts on the crown and spreads peripherally.

Dermoscopy of CCCA shows a preserved honeycomb pattern and pinpoint white dots with an irregular distribution. Depending on the severity of the disease, the affected scalp can be almost completely bald or show reduced hair density with miniaturized hairs and sparse terminal hairs emerging as single hairs or groups of two hairs surrounded by a peripilar grey–white halo. Irregular white patches corresponding to follicular scarring are scattered between the dots. Broken hairs and black dots can occasionally be seen. Erythema is common but the vascular pattern is not visible due to the presence of pigment.

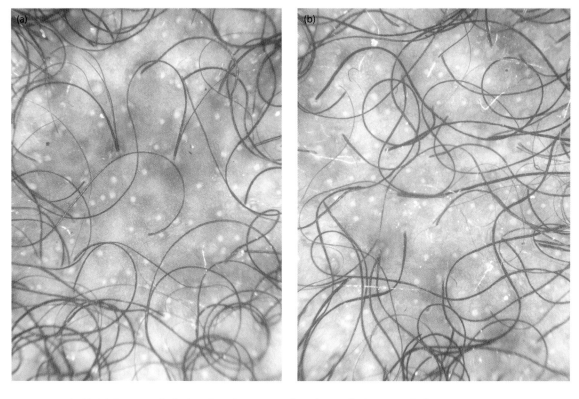

Figure 5.33 (a, b) CCCA: irregularly distributed pinpoint white dots and white–gray halos.

TRACTION ALOPECIA

Box 5.8 Traction Alopecia (Figures 5.34 through 5.36)

- More common in patients of African descent due to hairstyle habits.
- Scarring alopecia most commonly but not exclusively affects the marginal scalp.
- When the frontal and temporal scalp are affected, there is preservation of a rim of hairs at the hairline, called the "fringe sign."
- Dermoscopy: Loss of follicular openings/irregular pinpoint white dots, broken hairs, black dots, and persistence of vellus hairs.

Marginal traction alopecia is extremely common in women and children of African descent due to hair grooming practices and hairstyle preferences. However, it can be seen in all ethnicities. In its early phase, the alopecia is reversible, but it becomes permanent in longstanding disease.

Dermoscopy shows a loss of follicular openings or irregular pinpoint white dots in patients of color, irregular white patches corresponding to follicular scars, broken hairs, and black dots.

The presence of hair casts around the hair at the periphery of the patches indicates ongoing traction and suggests that the alopecia is likely to progress.

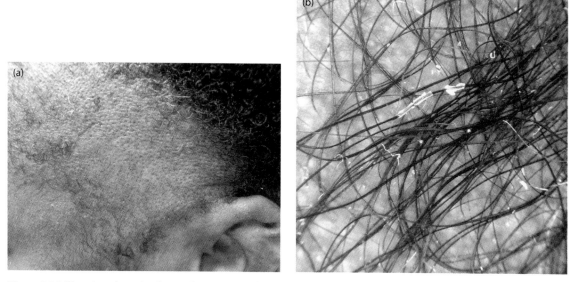

Figure 5.34 Traction alopecia: the patch is not complete bald. Also note the "fringe sign" consisting of a rim of hairs at the hairline (a). Dermoscopy at the periphery of the patch shows the presence of hair casts (b).

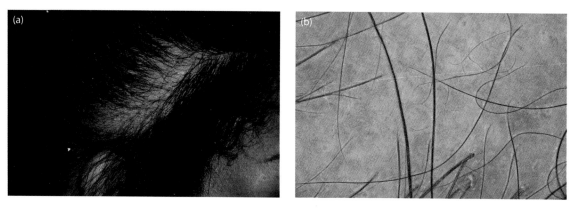

Figure 5.35 Traction alopecia: linear patch of alopecia due to hairstyle (a). Dermoscopy shows a loss of follicular openings. Vellus are preserved as they are too short to be pulled (b).

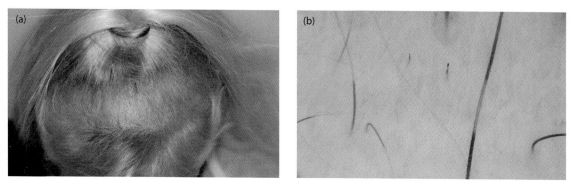

Figure 5.36 Traction alopecia: the patient is still wearing the traction hairstyle (a). Dermoscopy shows a loss of follicular openings and broken hairs (b). Vellus are preserved as they are too short to be pulled; yellow dots indicate follicular openings (c). *(Continued)*

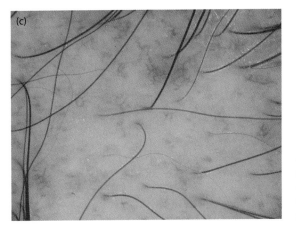

Figure 5.36 (Continued) Traction alopecia: the patient is still wearing the traction hairstyle (a). Dermoscopy shows a loss of follicular openings and broken hairs (b). Vellus are preserved as they are too short to be pulled; yellow dots indicate follicular openings (c).

SECONDARY SCARRING ALOPECIAS

Box 5.9 Secondary Scarring Alopecias (Figures 5.37 through 5.40)

- Alopecia is a feature of numerous conditions that involve the dermis and secondarily destroy the hair follicles.
- Dermoscopic features are not specific and only show loss of follicular openings.
- In erosive pustular dermatosis of the scalp, the hair roots are visible through the atrophic skin.

Secondary scarring alopecia is a feature of many disorders that cause a dermal scar and secondarily destroy the hair follicles. Dermoscopy can only help in establishing that there are no follicular openings and confirm whether it is a scarring alopecia. There are no features that enable the distinguishing of different causes of scarring alopecia at dermoscopy.

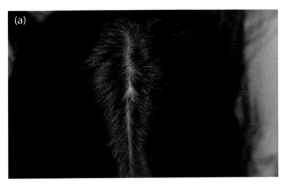
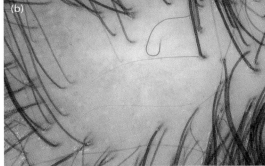

Figure 5.37 This 8-year-old child presents with a small patch of alopecia that has lasted for 5 months (a). Dermoscopy shows an absence of follicular openings (b). Possible diagnoses includes a scar from chickenpox or an insect bite.

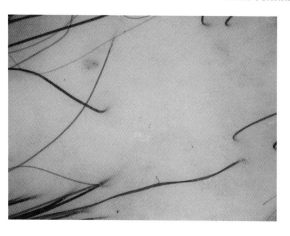

Figure 5.38 Dermoscopy of scarring alopecia due to a burn. Note the complete absence of follicular openings.

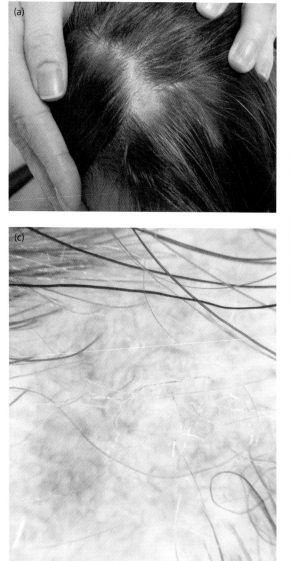

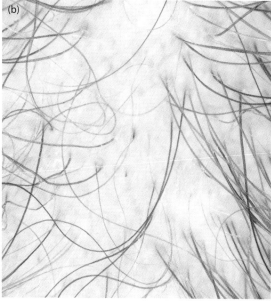

Figure 5.39 Scleroderma en coup de sabre (a). In early-stage disease, dermoscopy shows signs of nonscarring alopecia with broken hairs and black dots. However, the presence of peripilar casts and pili torti indicates a scarring process (b). In advanced-stage disease, dermoscopy shows a loss of follicular openings and arborizing vessels (c).

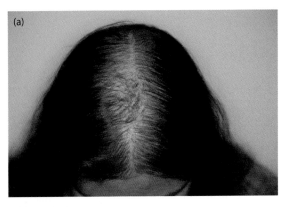

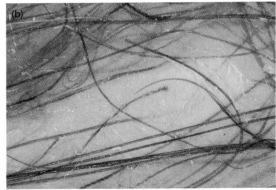

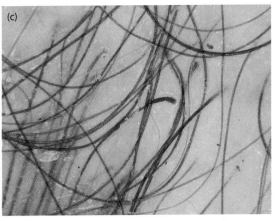

Figure 5.40 Erosive pustular dermatosis of the scalp (a). The scalp is so atrophic that it is possible to see the hair roots through the skin (b, c).

SUGGESTED READINGS

Duque-Estrada B, Tamler C, Sodré CT, Barcaui CB, Pereira FB. Dermoscopy patterns of cicatricial alopecia resulting from discoid lupus erythematosus and lichen planopilaris. *An Bras Dermatol.* 2010 Mar–Apr;85(2):179–83. Erratum in: *An Bras Dermatol.* 2010 Aug;85(4):578.

Fabris MR, Melo CP, Melo DF. Folliculitis decalvans: The use of dermatoscopy as an auxiliary tool in clinical diagnosis. *An Bras Dermatol.* 2013 Sep–Oct; 88(5):814–6.

Lacarrubba F, Micali G, Tosti A. Absence of vellus hair in the hairline: A videodermatoscopic feature of frontal fibrosing alopecia. *Br J Dermatol.* 2013 Aug;169(2):473–4.

Lanuti E, Miteva M, Romanelli P, Tosti A. Trichoscopy and histopathology of follicular keratotic plugs in scalp discoid lupus erythematosus. *Int J Trichol.* 2012 Jan;4(1):36–8.

Miteva M, Tosti A. Dermoscopy guided scalp biopsy in cicatricial alopecia. *J Eur Acad Dermatol Venereol.* 2013 Oct;27(10):1299–303.

Miteva M, Tosti A. Dermatoscopic features of central centrifugal cicatricial alopecia. *J Am Acad Dermatol.* 2014 Sep;71(3):443–9.

Pirmez R, Donati A, Valente NS, Sodré CT, Tosti A. Glabellar red dots in frontal fibrosing alopecia: A further clinical sign of vellus follicle involvement. *Br J Dermatol.* 2014 Mar;170(3):745–6.

Ross EK, Vincenzi C, Tosti A. Videodermoscopy in the evaluation of hair and scalp disorders. *J Am Acad Dermatol.* 2006 Nov;55(5):799–806.

Tosti A, Miteva M, Torres F, Vincenzi C, Romanelli P. Hair casts are a dermoscopic clue for the diagnosis of traction alopecia. *Br J Dermatol.* 2010 Dec; 163(6):1353–5.

Tosti A, Torres F, Misciali C, Vincenzi C, Starace M, Miteva M, Romanelli P. Follicular red dots: A novel dermoscopic pattern observed in scalp discoid lupus erythematosus. *Arch Dermatol.* 2009 Dec; 145(12):1406–9.

6 Hair shaft disorders
Antonella Tosti

Dermoscopy is a rapid and effective tool for diagnosing both congenital and acquired hair shaft disorders. It offers the great advantage of enabling the examination of a large number of hair shafts in a short period of time, including the eyebrows, eyelashes, and body hairs. This is very important as most shaft disorders involve a limited area of the scalp. In children, a painless and noninvasive way to rapidly examine the scalp and other hairs is crucial, as plucking or cutting the hair shafts is either painful or difficult in cases of short broken hairs. Most hair shaft disorders can be diagnosed by dermoscopy; the only exception is trichothiodystrophy. However, in trichothiodystrophy, dermoscopy can be useful in identifying the hairs that should be sampled for microscopic examination.

Box 6.1 Hair Shaft Disorders That Can Be Identified by Dermoscopy

- Monilethrix
- Pili torti
- Pili trianguli and canaliculi
- Pili annulati
- Trichorrhexis invaginata
- Trichorrhexis nodosa

MONILETHRIX

Box 6.2 Monilethrix (Figures 6.1 through 6.4)

- Alopecia resulting from hair shaft fragility.
- More severe in friction areas.
- Autosomal dominant (mutations in the human basic hair keratins hHb6 and hHb1).
- Autosomal recessive (rare and severe involving mutations in the desmoglein 4 gene).
- Follicular keratosis in the occipital region.
- Dermoscopy: Hair shaft beading, breakage at the internode level and affected hairs bending in different directions.

Monilethrix is a hair shaft disorder characterized by hair fragility with alopecia due to hair breakage.

The hair shaft has a beaded appearance due to the presence of elliptical nodes that are regularly separated by narrow internodes, which are the sites of fracture.

The alopecia is more severe on the scalp regions that are more exposed to friction, such as the occipital area, where the affected scalp also presents follicular keratosis.

The alopecia is present from childhood and the family history reveals other affected members, even though severity of the disease often varies between members of the same family. Hair fragility improves with age.

Dermoscopy reveals hair beading and breakage and confirms the diagnosis. The typical beading, characterized by elliptical nodes and intermittent constrictions at regular distances, is not limited to the scalp hair, but can also affect the eyebrows, eyelashes, or axilla. Breakage occurs at the internode level, where the medulla is absent. Affected hairs bend in different directions. Dermoscopy enables an evaluation of the severity of monilethrix as, in some patients, only a few hair shafts show the abnormality and breakage is minimal, whereas in other cases, most hair shafts, including vellus hairs, are affected and broken hairs are very numerous.

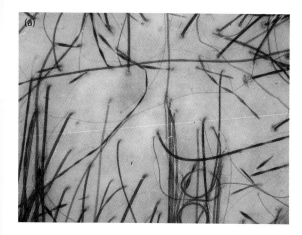

Figure 6.1 Monilethrix. Hair beading and breakage at different level from scalp emergence (a). Breakage occurs at the internode level (b). Note the absence of medulla at the internode level (c). *(Continued)*

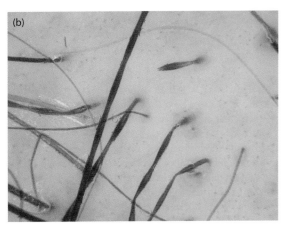
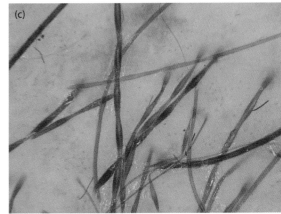

Figure 6.1 (*Continued*) Monilethrix. Hair beading and breakage at different level from scalp emergence (a). Breakage occurs at the internode level (b). Note the absence of medulla at the internode level (c).

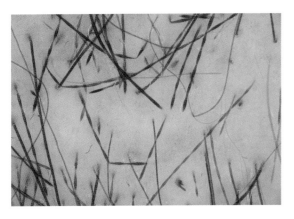

Figure 6.2 Monilethrix. Affected hairs bend in different directions.

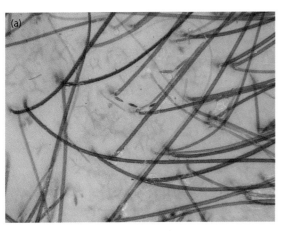
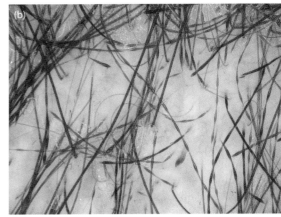

Figure 6.3 Monilethrix. Severity is variable, ranging from only very few hairs being affected (a), to the involvement of most hairs with moderate breakage (b), to the involvement of all scalp hair and the presence of small, broken, beaded fragments on the scalp surface (c). (*Continued*)

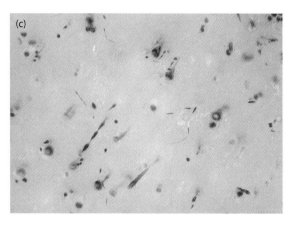

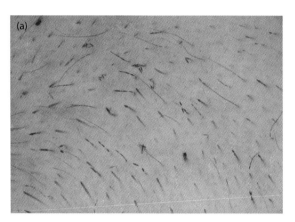

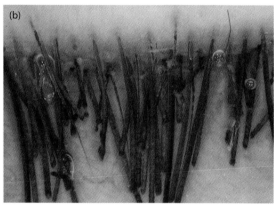

Figure 6.3 (Continued) Monilethrix. Severity is variable, ranging from only very few hairs being affected (a), to the involvement of most hairs with moderate breakage (b), to the involvement of all scalp hair and the presence of small, broken, beaded fragments on the scalp surface (c).

Figure 6.4 Monilethrix. The eyebrows show typical beading and breakage (a). The eyelashes show distal breakage and typical beading in a few vellus hairs (b).

PILI TORTI

Box 6.3 Pili Torti (Figures 6.5 and 6.6)

- Occasional finding in the normal scalp
- Common in patients with hair shaft disorders and genetic syndromes
- Common in scarring alopecias
- Dermoscopy: Flat and irregularly twisted shafts

A few pili torti can be occasionally observed in the normal scalp and are a very common finding in patients with cicatricial alopecia, particularly lichen planopilaris and frontal fibrosing alopecia. They are also seen in ectodermal dysplasias or in association with other hair shaft abnormalities.

Pili torti are a characteristic feature of Menkes and Bjornstad syndromes.

Dermoscopy shows a flattened hair shaft that twists through 180° at irregular intervals.

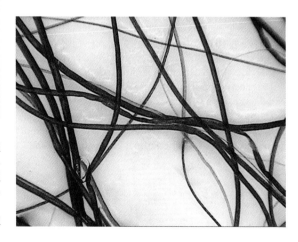

Figure 6.5 Pili torti: the hair shaft is flattened and irregularly twisted.

73

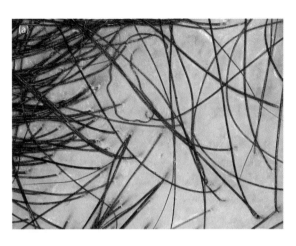

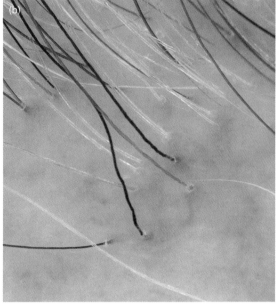

Figure 6.6 Pili torti are common in patients with scarring alopecias, such as lichen planopilaris (a) and frontal fibrosing alopecia (b).

PILI TRIANGULI AND CANALICULI (UNCOMBABLE HAIR)

> *Box 6.4* Pili Trianguli and Canaliculi (Figure 6.7)
>
> - Uncombable, dry, and unruly hair
> - Spontaneous improvement with aging
> - Dermoscopy: Triangular hair shafts with longitudinal grooving

Uncombable hair is characterized by dry, spun-glass, unruly hair that is impossible to comb. The condition affects children and improves spontaneously with aging.

The disorder may be inherited or sporadic.

Diagnosis of pili trianguli and canaliculi is usually based on scanning electron microscopy.

Dermoscopy is a valid and simple alternative. The hair shaft has a triangular or reniform shape and, in most cases, presents with a longitudinal groove or flattening.

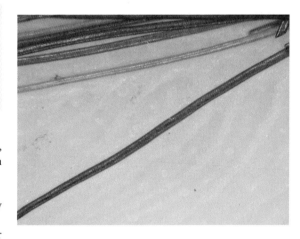

Figure 6.7 Triangular hair shaft with a longitudinal groove.

PILI ANNULATI

Pili annulati is an autosomal dominant hair shaft abnormality characterized by a speckled, shiny appearance of the hair.

The hair shafts present air-filled cavities that appear as light bands along their lengths. The condition is not associated with hair fragility, but the affected hair is more susceptible to weathering.

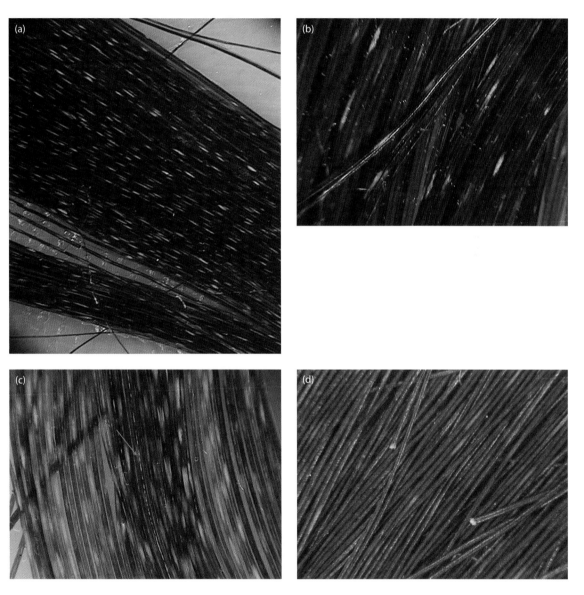

Figure 6.8 Pili annulati: the white bands correspond to air-filled cavities within the hair cortex (a, b). The white bands should not be confused with the medulla (arrow), which is also visible as small interrupted bands in the hair shaft (c). Trichorrhexis nodosa and pili annulati (d).

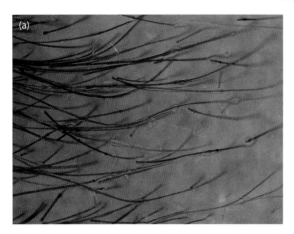
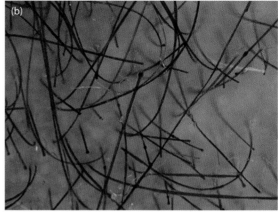

Figure 6.9 (a, b) Trichorrhexis invaginata: the hair shafts show single or multiple ball-shaped nodes at irregular intervals. Hair breakage mostly occurs in correspondence to the knots: the golf-tea sign. Also note the broken shafts with a ragged cupped shape (a, b). (Courtesy of Laila El Shabrawi, MD, Austria.)

TRICHORRHEXIS INVAGINATA (BAMBOO HAIR)

Box 6.6 Trichorrhexis Invaginata (Bamboo Hair) (Figure 6.9)

- Alopecia resulting from hair shaft fragility.
- More severe in friction areas.
- Typical of Netherton disease, a rare autosomal recessive genodermatosis that combines ichthyosis, bamboo hair, and atopic dermatitis.
- The hair shaft shows multiple knots along its length.
- Dermoscopy: Hair shaft breakage and hair shaft knots.

In trichorrhexis invaginata, the hair shaft shows multiple knots along its length. The knots consists of a proximal cup-shaped portion and a distal ball-shaped portion, resembling the ball-and-cup joint of bamboo. Hair breakage mostly affects the scalp areas exposed to friction.

The alopecia may be severe. This hair shaft disorder frequently affects the eyelashes and eyebrows, which may present the abnormality even when the scalp hair—which improves with age—appears normal.

Trichorrhexis invaginata is a feature of Netherton disease, a rare autosomal recessive genodermatosis that combines ichthyosis, bamboo hair, and atopic dermatitis.

At dermoscopy, the hair shaft shows nodular swellings at irregular intervals. Ball-shaped knots similar to matchsticks and hair breakage are evident.

TRICHORRHEXIS NODOSA

Box 6.7 Trichorrhexis Nodosa

- Acquired hair shaft disorder.
- Most common sign of hair weathering.
- Hair shaft shows white knots and fractures.
- Dermoscopy: Brush-like hair fracturing (see Chapter 10).

SUGGESTED READINGS

Burk C, Hu S, Lee C, Connelly EA. Netherton syndrome and trichorrhexis invaginata—A novel diagnostic approach. *Pediatr Dermatol.* 2008 Mar–Apr;25(2):287–8.

Lencastre A, Tosti A. Monilethrix. *J Pediatr.* 2012 Dec; 161(6):1176.

Lencastre A, Tosti A. Role of trichoscopy in children's scalp and hair disorders. *Pediatr Dermatol.* 2013;30(6):674–82.

Miteva M, Tosti A. Dermatoscopy of hair shaft disorders. *J Am Acad Dermatol.* 2013 Mar;68(3):473–81.

Rakowska A, Kowalska-Oledzka E, Slowinska M, Rosinska D, Rudnicka L. Hair shaft videodermoscopy in Netherton syndrome. *Pediatr Dermatol.* 2009 May–Jun;26(3):320–2.

Rakowska A, Slowinska M, Kowalska-Oledzka E, Rudnicka L. Trichoscopy in genetic hair shaft abnormalities. *J Dermatol Case Rep.* 2008 Jul;2(2):14–20.

Rudnicka L, Rakowska A, Kerzeja M, Olszewska M. Hair shafts in trichoscopy: Clues for diagnosis of hair and scalp diseases. *Dermatol Clin.* 2013 Oct;31(4):695–708.

Silverberg NB, Silverberg JI, Wong ML. Trichoscopy using a handheld dermoscope: An in-office technique to diagnose genetic disease of the hair. *Arch Dermatol.* 2009 May;145(5):600–1.

7 Pediatric hair disorders
Antonella Tosti

APLASIA CUTIS CONGENITA

Box 7.1 Aplasia Cutis Congenita (Figure 7.1)

- Present from birth
- Localized patch of alopecia with an atrophic surface
- Dermoscopy: Loss of follicular openings

SEBACEOUS NEVUS

Box 7.2 Sebaceous Nevus (Figures 7.2 through 7.4)

- Present since birth.
- Localized yellowish patch of alopecia in infancy.
- Alopecic patch with verrucoid appearance after puberty.
- Dermoscopy: Bright yellow spots not associated with follicular structures in infancy. Yellow lobular-like structures surrounded by small vessels after puberty. Dermoscopy is helpful for detecting basal cell carcinomas arising on sebaceous nevi.

The condition is rare, affecting 3/10,000 newborns. The scalp is involved in most cases with a round or oval patch of variable size of hair loss, characterized by atrophic skin. A defect in the underlying bone may be associated. At dermoscopy, the patch has a translucent appearance and shows an absence of follicular openings. Hair roots can be visible through the skin at the periphery of the patch. Dermoscopy is very useful for distinguishing aplasia cutis from sebaceous nevus in newborns.

Sebaceous nevus is a common congenital lesion that is generally first noticed at birth. Before puberty, sebaceous nevi appear as well-demarcated plaques of yellowish color with alopecia. After puberty, the patch becomes verrucoid and micronodular and changes in color from yellow to dark brown. Tumors, including basal cell carcinomas, may arise in sebaceous nevi.

In infancy, dermoscopy shows bright yellow spots that are not associated with follicular structures. After puberty, sebaceous nevi are characterized by yellow lobular-like structures surrounded by small vessels. Dermoscopy is helpful for detecting basal cell carcinomas arising on sebaceous nevi.

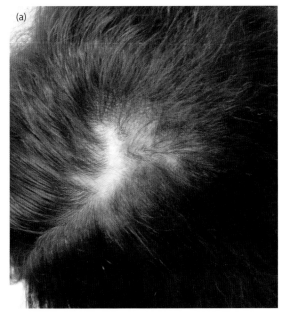

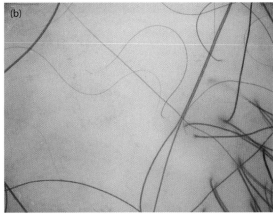

Figure 7.1 (a) Aplasia cutis congenita. (b) Dermoscopy shows loss of follicular openings, and a visible anagen root.

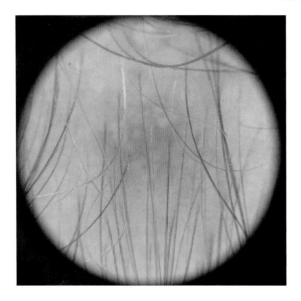

Figure 7.2 Sebaceous nevus in a newborn. Dermoscopy shows bright yellow spots not associated with follicular structures. (Courtesy of Dr. Iria Neri, Bologna, Italy.)

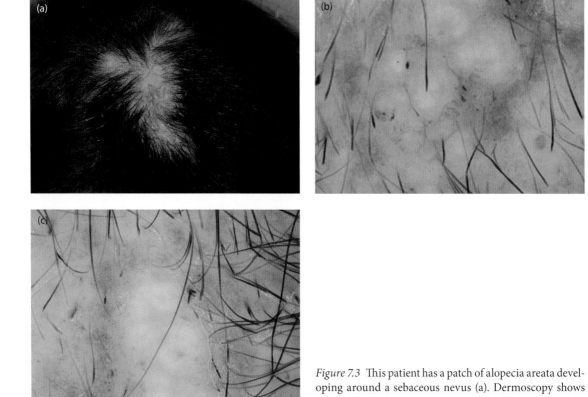

Figure 7.3 This patient has a patch of alopecia areata developing around a sebaceous nevus (a). Dermoscopy shows yellow lobular-like structures surrounded by small vessels; typical features of alopecia areata are also present (b, c).

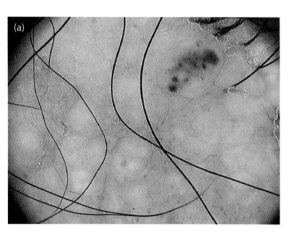

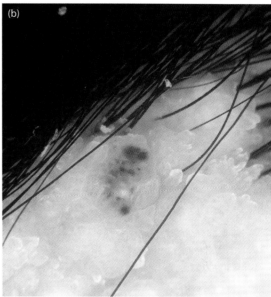

Figure 7.4 Basal cell carcinoma on a sebaceous nevus. Dermoscopy shows yellow lobular-like structures, and the presence of blue–gray ovoid nests at the periphery of the lesions suggesting the diagnosis of basal cell carcinoma (a, b), which was confirmed by pathology.

CONGENITAL TRIANGULAR ALOPECIA

Box 7.3 Congenital Triangular Alopecia (Figures 7.5 and 7.6)

- Triangular or oval patch on the temporal scalp.
- Often noticed after 5 years of age.
- The patch contains vellus hair follicles.
- Dermoscopy shows a carpet of vellus hairs surrounded by terminal hairs.

This condition is not rare and is usually diagnosed in childhood. A triangular or oval patch of alopecia is observed in the temporal region. The condition may be bilateral.

The area contains fine vellus hair and remains stable over time.

Dermoscopy is useful for ruling out alopecia areata or scarring alopecia when the patch has an atypical location. The bald area contains numerous vellus hairs and yellow dots are absent.

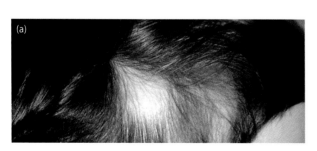

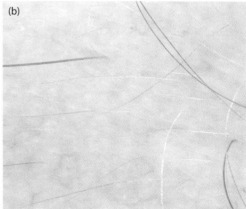

Figure 7.5 (a, b) Congenital triangular alopecia in a child. Dermoscopy reveals fine vellus hairs. Yellow dots are not present.

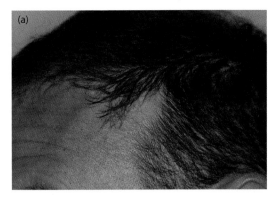

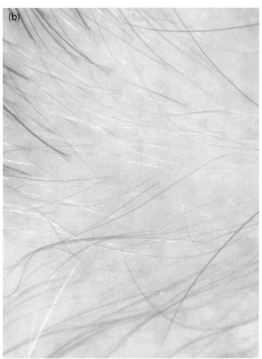

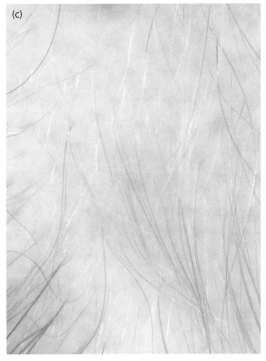

Figure 7.6 Congenital triangular alopecia in an adult (a). Dermoscopy of the patch reveals a carpet of vellus hairs (b) surrounded by terminal hairs at the patch's periphery (c).

LOOSE ANAGEN HAIR SYNDROME

Box 7.4 Loose Anagen Hair Syndrome (Figure 7.7)

- Hair that does not grow long and patches of alopecia.
- Easily and painlessly pluckable hair.
- Diagnosis is based on the presence of anagen hairs devoid of sheaths (loose anagen hairs) at pull test and trichogram.
- Dermoscopy of the scalp is not specific. It is useful for evaluating the hair roots.

The loose anagen hair syndrome is a sporadic or familial hair disorder that primarily affects children. The condition is due to a defective anchorage of the hair shaft to the follicle, resulting in easily and painlessly pluckable hair. Patients complain that the hair does not grow long. Hair density can be normal or reduced and irregular bald patches due to traumatic painless extraction of hair tufts can be present. The hair may be dull and unruly. Diagnosis is based on clinical features and the presence of anagen hairs devoid of sheaths at pull test and trichogram.

Dermoscopy of the scalp is not specific. It may be useful for evaluating the hairs extracted with the pull test.

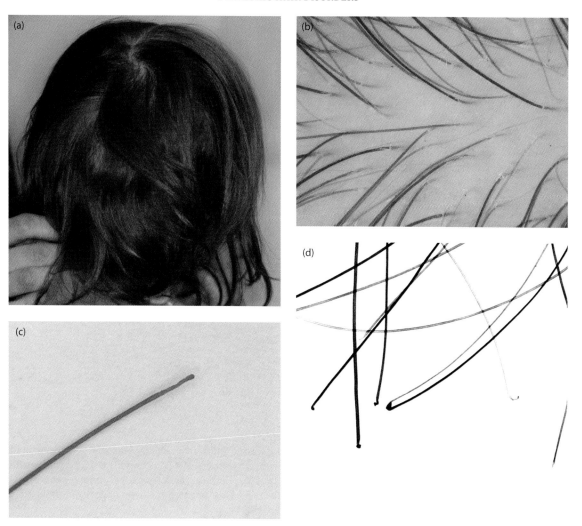

Figure 7.7 Loose anagen hair syndrome. Short hair and a small alopecic patch (a). Dermoscopy shows normal hair density and thickness (b). Dermoscopy of the hair obtained with the pull test shows an anagen hair devoid of a sheath (c). The diagnosis was confirmed by trichogram (d).

SHORT ANAGEN HAIR SYNDROME

Box 7.5 Short Anagen Hair Syndrome (Figure 7.8)

- Very short hair and relapsing episodes of telogen effluvium.
- Dermoscopy of the scalp is not specific. Dermoscopy of the pulled hairs shows short (less than 6 cm long) telogen hairs with tipped points.

In this condition, hair is very short. Hair shortness is due to the short duration of the anagen phase and not to slow hair growth. Relapsing episodes of telogen effluvium are also typical. Diagnosis is confirmed by the pull test that shows short (less than 6 cm long) telogen hairs with tipped points.

Dermoscopy of the scalp is not specific. Dermoscopy of the pulled hairs is a fast method of confirming that the root is in telogen and that the tip has not been cut.

81

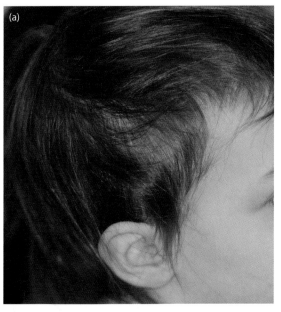

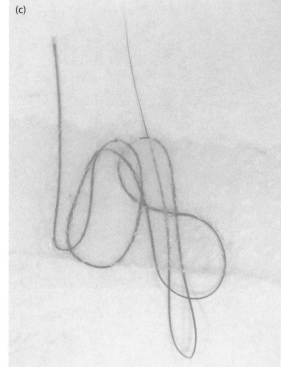

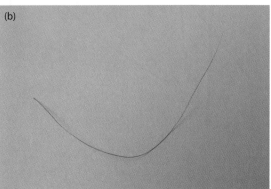

Figure 7.8 Short anagen hair syndrome. Very short hair with reduced density (a). The pull test is positive with short hairs less than 6 cm long (b). Dermoscopy allows for the rapid assessment of the root (telogen) and the pointed tip (c).

TRAUMATIC ALOPECIA

Box 7.6 Traumatic Alopecia (Figure 7.9)

- Acute alopecia can occur after scalp traumas.
- Patchy alopecia that is likely induced by pressure.

- Dermoscopy shows features similar to alopecia areata.

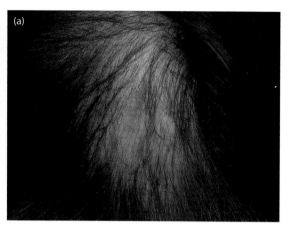
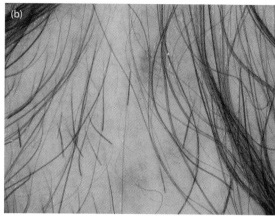

Figure 7.9 This child developed an area of alopecia after closure of a scalp wound with glue (a). Dermoscopy shows features that resemble alopecia areata with broken and exclamation mark hairs (b).

SUGGESTED READINGS

Iorizzo M, Pazzaglia M, Starace M, Militello G, Tosti A. Videodermoscopy: A useful tool for diagnosing congenital triangular alopecia. *Pediatr Dermatol.* 2008 Nov–Dec;25(6):652–4.

Lacarrubba F, Micali G. Congenital triangular alopecia. *BMJ Case Rep.* 2014 Jan 8.

Lencastre A, Tosti A. Role of trichoscopy in children's scalp and hair disorders. *Pediatr Dermatol.* 2013;30(6):674–82.

Neri I, Savoia F, Giacomini F, Raone B, Aprile S, Patrizi A. Usefulness of dermatoscopy for the early diagnosis of sebaceous naevus and differentiation from aplasia cutis congenita. *Clin Exp Dermatol.* 2009 Jul;34(5):e50–2.

8 Dermoscopy of the black scalp
Antonella Tosti

NONSCARRING VERSUS SCARRING ALOPECIAS

Box 8.1 Nonscarring versus Scarring Alopecias
(Figures 8.1 and 8.2)

- Nonscarring: Regular pinpoint white dots
- Scarring: Irregular pinpoint white dots and white patches

The presence of pinpoint white dots makes distinguishing scarring from nonscarring alopecia more difficult than in the nonpigmented scalp, as the loss of follicular openings is not immediately evident. In nonscarring alopecias, the dot distribution is very regular and dots often contain miniaturized or broken hair shafts. In scarring alopecia, the pinpoint white dots have an irregular distribution, as the dots corresponding to the follicular openings are no longer present. The follicular scars appear as white patches.

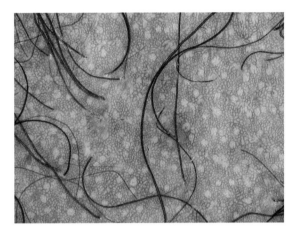

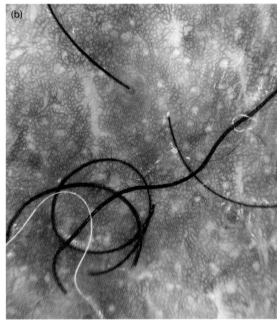

Figure 8.1 Nonscarring alopecia: numerous pinpoint white dots with a regular distribution.

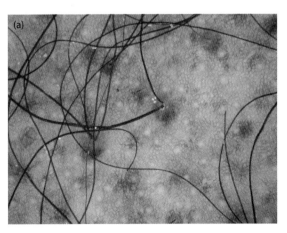

Figure 8.2 Scarring alopecia: the pinpoint white dots are irregularly distributed (a). Severe scarring alopecia: irregular pinpoint white dots and white patches (b).

ANDROGENETIC ALOPECIA

Box 8.2 Androgenetic Alopecia (Figure 8.3)

- More than 20% variability in the hair shaft diameter
- Presence of short, thin (0.03 mm in diameter) regrowing hairs in the frontal scalp

The prevalence of androgenetic alopecia in patients of African descent is lower than in Caucasians and a differential diagnosis with central centrifugal cicatricial alopecia may be difficult. The alopecic area shows a preserved honeycomb pattern and regularly distributed pinpoint white dots.

The criteria for diagnosis are the same as for Caucasians.

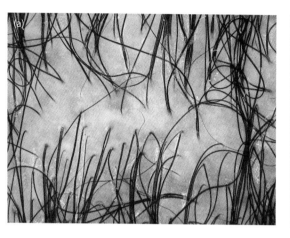 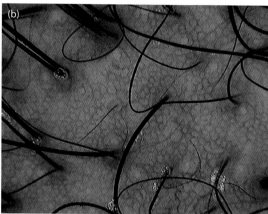

Figure 8.3 Androgenetic alopecia. More than 20% variability in the hair shaft diameter (a). Short, thin regrowing hairs in the frontal scalp (b).

ALOPECIA AREATA

Box 8.3 Alopecia Areata (Figures 8.4 and 8.5)

- Regular pinpoint white dots
- Exclamation mark hairs, broken hairs, black dots, and circle hairs

The alopecic patches show the honeycomb pattern and pinpoint white dots. Diagnosis is based on the presence of exclamation mark hairs, broken hairs, black dots, and circle hairs.

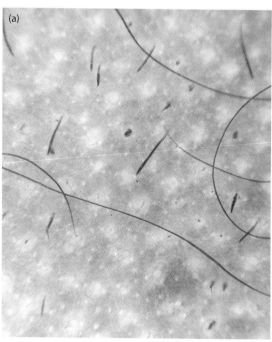

Figure 8.4 Alopecia areata: pinpoint white dots with a regular distribution. Presence of exclamation mark hairs (a), broken hairs and black dots (b), and circle hairs (c). *(Continued)*

(b)

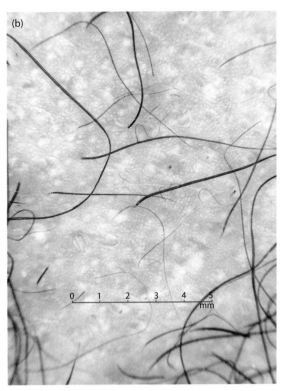

(c)

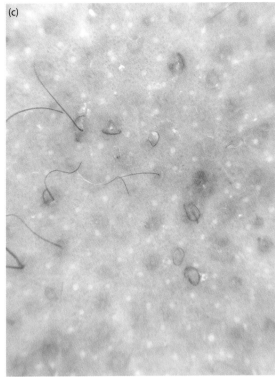

Figure 8.4 (*Continued*) Alopecia areata: pinpoint white dots with a regular distribution. Presence of exclamation mark hairs (a), broken hairs and black dots (b), and circle hairs (c).

Figure 8.5 Alopecia areata totalis: regular pinpoint white dots.

ALOPECIA DUE TO HAIR BREAKAGE

Box 8.4 Alopecia due to Hair Breakage (Figure 8.6)

- Affected scalp areas show a normal hair density.
- Trichorrhexis nodosa, trichoptilosis, and brush-like ends in the shafts obtained with the tug test.

African hair is very delicate and therefore highly susceptible to mechanical, physical, and chemical damage.

Diffuse or patchy alopecia due to hair breakage is a common disease in women. Patients often do not correlate the hair problem with their styling procedures and either complain of alopecia or that their hair does not grow long. Scalp dermoscopy reveals a preserved honeycomb pattern and regularly distributed pinpoint white dots. The hair density in affected scalp areas is not reduced as compared with unaffected areas. Broken hairs may be difficult to detect. Diagnosis is very easy and fast by performing dermoscopy on the hairs obtained via the tug test. These show longitudinal fissuring, knots, and brush-like ends due to trichorrhexis nodosa.

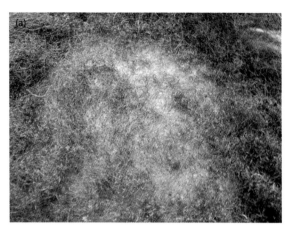

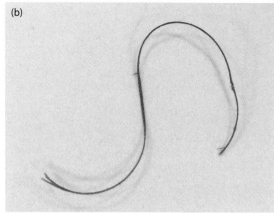

Figure 8.6 Patchy alopecia due to hair breakage (a). Dermoscopy of the hair shafts extracted with the tug test shows focal knots with initial breakage, longitudinal fissuring, and a brush-like tip (b).

TINEA CAPITIS

Box 8.5 Tinea Capitis (Figures 8.7 and 8.8)

- Corkscrew hairs
- Comma hairs
- Black dots, hair casts, and pustules

Corkscrew hairs are a characteristic dermoscopic finding of tinea capitis in black children and adults. These appear as irregularly twisted short hairs and are usually seen in association with the broken, comma-shaped hairs that characterize tinea capitis in Caucasians. Corkscrew hairs are exclusive to African-descent patients, where they are seen both in endothrix and ectothrix infections. Their shape is likely linked to the anatomical shape of African hairs. Pustules, broken hairs, black dots, and hair casts are also observed.

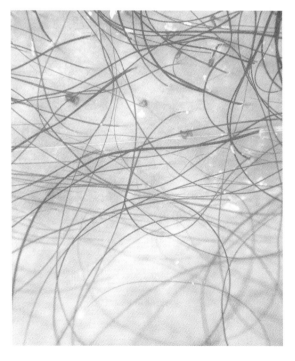

Figure 8.7 Tinea capitis: corkscrew hairs.

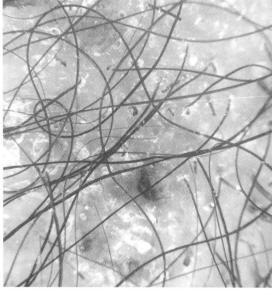

Figure 8.8 Tinea capitis, kerion: intense erythema, and scaling. Diagnostic features include comma hairs and corkscrew hairs. Black dots and broken hairs with casts are also evident.

TRACTION ALOPECIA

Marginal traction alopecia is extremely common in women and children of African descent due to hair-grooming practices and hairstyle preferences. In its early phase, the alopecia is reversible, but it becomes permanent in the longstanding disease. Dermoscopy of early-stage disease shows a preserved honeycomb pattern and regularly distributed pinpoint white dots. The hair density is reduced, with numerous miniaturized hairs. Severe traction can cause elongation and linearization of follicular ostia.

In advanced-stage disease, the pinpoint white dots show an irregular distribution and the follicular scars become evident as irregular white patches.

It is important to evaluate the hairs along the hairline at the periphery of the alopecia for hair casts. These appear as small, mobile, spindle-edged, white-to-brown cylindrical structures that surround the proximal hair shaft. Their presence indicates ongoing traction and suggests that the alopecia is likely to progress. Dermoscopy can then establish whether the hairstyle is still causing traction, which is very important, as long-term traction leads to permanent scarring.

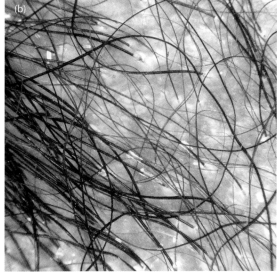

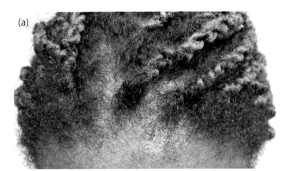

Figure 8.9 Early traction alopecia (a). The presence of hair casts along the hair shafts at the periphery of the patch confirms that the hairstyle is causing the traction (b).

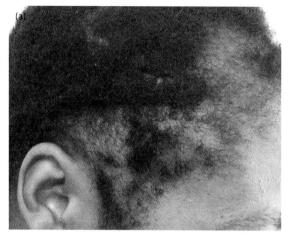

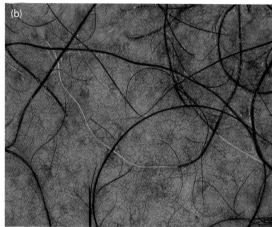

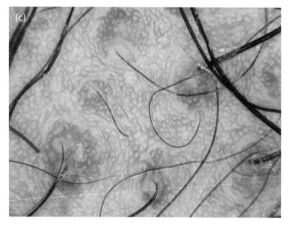

Figure 8.10 Longstanding traction alopecia (a). Dermoscopy shows reduced hair density with numerous miniaturized hairs (b). At high magnification, it is possible to detect hair breakage (c).

DISSECTING CELLULITIS

Box 8.8 Dissecting Cellulitis (Figure 8.11)

- Enlarged plugged follicular openings
- Black dots and broken hairs

Dissecting cellulitis is a rare scalp disease seen mostly in young males of Afro-American or Hispanic descent. The disease is characterized by perifollicular pustules, painful suppurative nodules, and fluctuating abscesses, as well as by intercommunicating sinus tracts on the scalp.

Dermatoscopy of the alopecic patches overlying the painful nodules shows a pattern of nonscarring alopecia. The honeycomb pattern is preserved and the alopecic area shows regularly distributed pinpoint white dots, enlarged plugged follicular openings, black dots, and broken hairs.

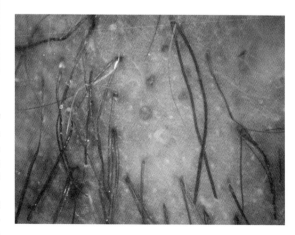

Figure 8.11 Dissecting cellulitis: dermoscopy of the alopecic patch shows pinpoint white dots, enlarged plugged follicular openings, black dots, and broken hairs.

CENTRAL CENTRIFUGAL CICATRICIAL ALOPECIA

Central centrifugal cicatricial alopecia (CCCA) is a common scarring alopecia that exclusively affects women of African descent. It is characterized by an area of permanent hair loss that involves the crown and vertex and spreads centrifugally over time.

Dermoscopy of CCCA shows a preserved honeycomb pattern and pinpoint white dots with an irregular distribution. Depending on the severity of the disease, the affected scalp can be almost completely bald or show reduced hair density, with miniaturized hairs and sparse terminal hairs emerging as single hairs or groups of two hairs surrounded by a peripilar gray–white halo. Irregular white patches corresponding to follicular scarring are scattered between the dots. Broken hairs and black dots can occasionally be seen. In the sun-exposed scalp, the pigmentation often shows a fingertip pattern with pigmented asterisk-like macules.

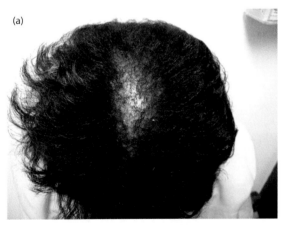

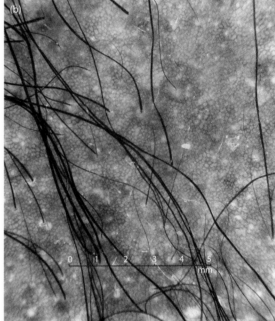

Figure 8.12 CCCA (a). Dermoscopy shows irregularly distributed pinpoint white dots, irregular white patches, miniaturized hairs, and terminal hairs with a peripilar white–gray halo (b).

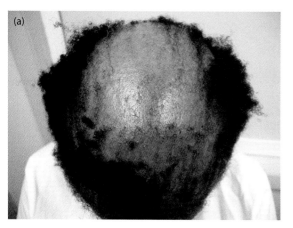

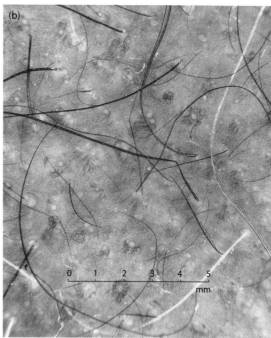

Figure 8.13 Severe CCCA (a). Dermoscopy shows irregular pinpoint white dots, irregular white patches, miniaturized hairs, and few remaining terminal hairs surrounded by a white–gray halo (b).

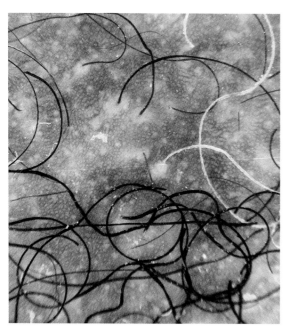

Figure 8.14 CCCA: white–gray halos associated with broken hairs.

LICHEN PLANOPILARIS

Box 8.10 Lichen Planopilaris (Figures 8.15 through 8.17)

- Irregularly distributed pinpoint white dots and irregular white patches
- Peripilar casts
- Perifollicular blue–gray dots with a target pattern

Lichen planopilaris is uncommon in patients of African descent. Dermoscopy shows a preserved honeycomb pattern with irregularly distributed pinpoint white dots. The alopecic areas present irregular white patches and peripilar casts around the terminal hairs within and surrounding the patches. Perifollicular blue–gray dots with an annular or "target" pattern are occasionally seen and pathologically correspond to melanin particles within melanophages or the papillary dermis. The target pattern corresponds to the distribution of the follicles that have been destroyed by the disease.

91

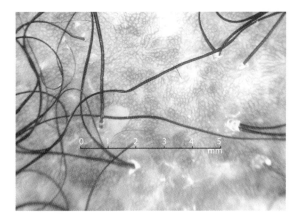

Figure 8.15 Lichen planopilaris: the alopecic area shows irregular white patches. The hairs at the periphery of the patch show thick peripilar casts.

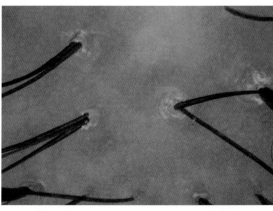

Figure 8.16 Lichen planopilaris: peripilar casts and hair tufting.

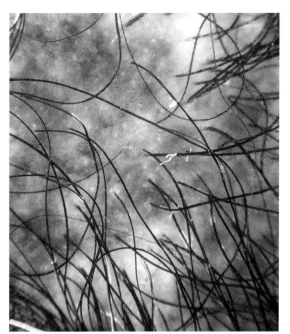

Figure 8.17 Lichen planopilaris: perifollicular blue–gray dots with annular or "target" pattern.

FRONTAL FIBROSING ALOPECIA

Box 8.11 Frontal Fibrosing Alopecia (Figures 8.18 through 8.19)

- Irregularly distributed pinpoint white dots and irregular white patches
- Peripilar casts
- Loss of vellus hair at the hairline

Its frequent association with traction alopecia complicates the diagnosis of frontal fibrosing alopecia in women of African descent.

At dermoscopy, the new hairline is devoid of vellus hairs and shows terminal hairs with peripilar casts, which may be subtle or very prominent. Black dots and broken hairs can also be seen. The alopecic scalp shows the pinpoint white dot pattern and white patches. Frontal fibrosing alopecia in dark phototypes is frequently associated with facial papules and lichen pigmentosus.

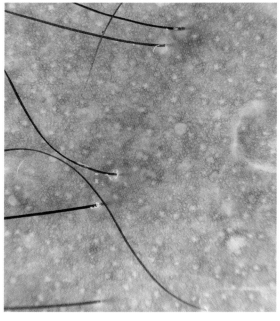

Figure 8.18 Frontal fibrosing alopecia: absence of vellus hairs and presence of peripilar casts at emergence of the hair shafts along the hairline.

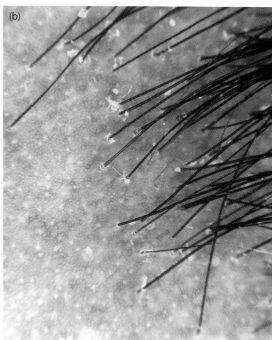

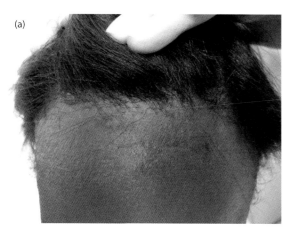

Figure 8.19 Frontal fibrosing alopecia with facial papules and lichen pigmentosus (a). Dermoscopy shows the absence of vellus hairs and prominent peripilar casts (b).

DISCOID LUPUS ERYTHEMATOSUS

Box 8.12 Discoid Lupus Erythematosus (Figures 8.20 through 8.22)

- Loss of pigmentation with disruption of the honeycomb pattern
- Follicular keratotic plugs
- Red dots
- Giant irregular capillaries
- Perifollicular and interfollicular blue–gray dots with a speckled pattern

Discoid lupus erythematosus is quite common in patients of African descent. Dermoscopy shows disruption of the honeycomb pattern with a loss of pigmentation within the alopecic areas. Pinpoint white dots are reduced or absent, with evident scarring.

Dermoscopic features include: loss of the pigmented honeycomb pattern with red dots, loss of the pigmented honeycomb pattern with follicular keratotic plugs, and the presence of giant tortuous capillaries.

Blue–gray dots, when present, show a speckled pattern, as the pigment incontinence is not limited to the follicles, but it also involves the interfollicular epidermis.

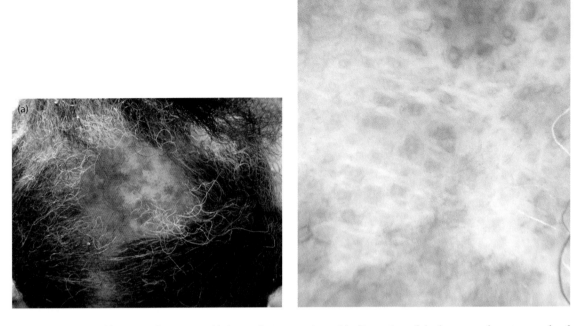

Figure 8.20 Discoid lupus erythematosus (a). Loss of pigmentation with disruption of the honeycomb pattern and red dots (b).

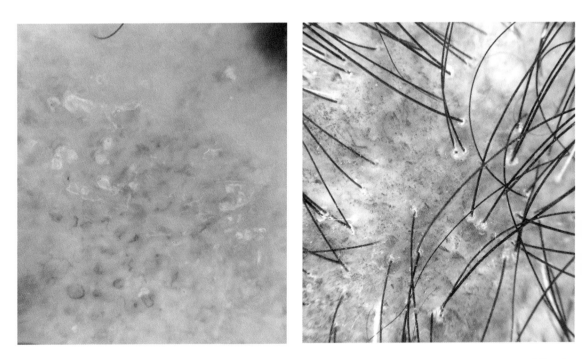

Figure 8.21 Discoid lupus erythematosus: loss of the pigmentation with disruption of the honeycomb pattern, keratotic follicular plugs, and giant irregular capillaries.

Figure 8.22 Discoid lupus erythematosus: perifollicular and interfollicular blue–gray dots with a speckled pattern.

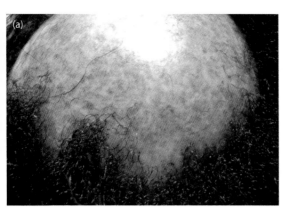
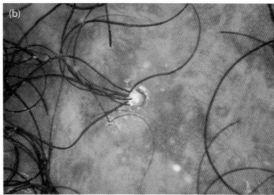

Figure 8.23 Folliculitis decalvans (a). Dermoscopy shows focal disruption of the honeycomb pattern, irregularly distributed pinpoint white dots and hair tufting with peripilar scales (b).

FOLLICULITIS DECALVANS

Box 8.13 Folliculitis Decalvans (Figure 8.23)

- Loss of pigmentation with disruption of the honeycomb pattern
- Tufts of six or more hairs emerging together

Folliculitis decalvans is uncommon in patients of African descent. Dermoscopy of the alopecic patch shows focal disruption of the honeycomb pattern with loss of pigmentation. The pinpoint white dots are reduced in number and irregularly interspersed with irregular white patches. The periphery of the patch shows tufts of six or more hairs emerging together, often associated with scalp erythema.

PEARLS FOR THE CLINICIANS

The black scalp has unique characteristics that make the diagnosis of hair and scalp disorders more difficult at dermoscopy. It is important to keep in mind that some diseases, such as traction alopecia and CCCA, are very common in women of African ancestry because of the intrinsic characteristics of their hair and their styling procedures. The existence of two or even three different hair disorders in the same patient is not rare, and dermoscopy is very important to the clinician by showing the specific features of the different conditions (Figures 8.24 and 8.25).

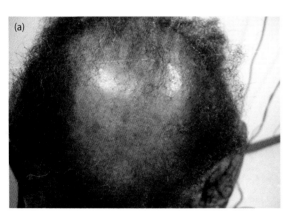
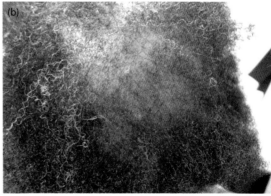

Figure 8.24 This patient has been affected by alopecia of the vertex for many years (a) and complains of recent patches of hair loss in the parietal and occipital scalp (b). Dermoscopy of the patch of the vertex shows irregular pinpoint white dots, irregular white patches, and terminal hairs surrounded by a white–gray halo (c). Dermoscopy of the parietal and occipital patches show comma hairs and black dots (d). The diagnosis of CCCA associated with tinea capitis was confirmed by cultures and pathology. *(Continued)*

95

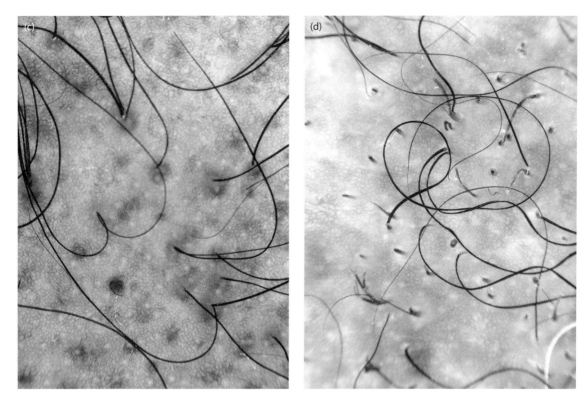

Figure 8.24 (*Continued*) This patient has been affected by alopecia of the vertex for many years (a) and complains of recent patches of hair loss in the parietal and occipital scalp (b). Dermoscopy of the patch of the vertex shows irregular pinpoint white dots, irregular white patches, and terminal hairs surrounded by a white–gray halo (c). Dermoscopy of the parietal and occipital patches show comma hairs and black dots (d). The diagnosis of CCCA associated with tinea capitis was confirmed by cultures and pathology.

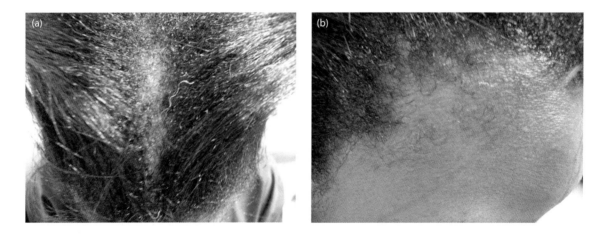

Figure 8.25 This patient has been affected by alopecia of the vertex for many years (a) and complains of a recent patches of hair loss in the temporal scalp (b). Dermoscopy of the patch of the vertex shows irregular pinpoint white dots, irregular white patches, and terminal hairs surrounded by a white–gray halo (c). Dermoscopy of the temporal patch shows regular pinpoint white dots, black dots, and broken hairs (d). The diagnosis of CCCA associated with alopecia areata was confirmed by pathology. (*Continued*)

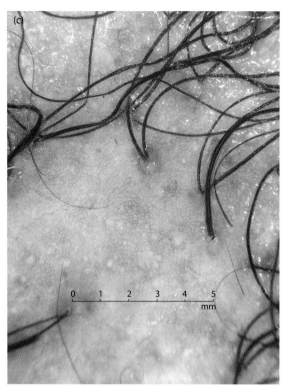
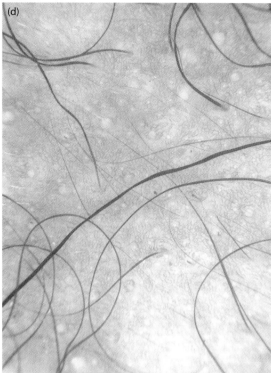

Figure 8.25 (*Continued*) This patient has been affected by alopecia of the vertex for many years (a) and complains of a recent patches of hair loss in the temporal scalp (b). Dermoscopy of the patch of the vertex shows irregular pinpoint white dots, irregular white patches, and terminal hairs surrounded by a white–gray halo (c). Dermoscopy of the temporal patch shows regular pinpoint white dots, black dots, and broken hairs (d). The diagnosis of CCCA associated with alopecia areata was confirmed by pathology.

SUGGESTED READINGS

Abraham LS, Piñeiro-Maceira J, Duque-Estrada B, Barcaui CB, Sodré CT. Pinpoint white dots in the scalp: Dermoscopic and histopathologic correlation. *J Am Acad Dermatol.* 2010 Oct;63(4):721–2.

de Moura LH, Duque-Estrada B, Abraham LS, Barcaui CB, Sodre CT. Dermoscopy findings of alopecia areata in an African-American patient. *J Dermatol Case Rep.* 2008 Dec;2(4):52–4.

Duque-Estrada B, Tamler C, Sodré CT, Barcaui CB, Pereira FB. Dermoscopy patterns of cicatricial alopecia resulting from discoid lupus erythematosus and lichen planopilaris. *An Bras Dermatol.* 2010 Mar–Apr;85(2):179–83. Erratum in: *An Bras Dermatol.* 2010 Aug;85(4):578.

Hughes R, Chiaverini C, Bahadoran P, Lacour JP. Corkscrew hair: A new dermoscopic sign for diagnosis of tinea capitis in black children. *Arch Dermatol.* 2011 Mar;147(3):355–6.

Miteva M, Tosti A. Hair and scalp dermatoscopy. *J Am Acad Dermatol.* 2012 Nov;67(5):1040–8.

Miteva M, Tosti A. Dermatoscopic features of central centrifugal cicatricial alopecia. *J Am Acad Dermatol.* 2014 Sep;71(3):443–9.

Miteva M, Whiting D, Harries M, Bernardes A, Tosti A. Frontal fibrosing alopecia in black patients. *Br J Dermatol.* 2012 Jul;167(1):208–10.

Pinheiro AM, Lobato LA, Varella TC. Dermoscopy findings in tinea capitis: Case report and literature review. *An Bras Dermatol.* 2012 Mar–Apr;87(2):313–4.

Tosti A, Miteva M, Torres F, Vincenzi C, Romanelli P. Hair casts are a dermoscopic clue for the diagnosis of traction alopecia. *Br J Dermatol.* 2010 Dec;163(6):1353–5.

Tosti A, Torres F, Miteva M. Dermoscopy of early dissecting cellulitis of the scalp simulates alopecia areata. *Actas Dermosifiliogr.* 2013 Jan;104(1):92–3.

Yin NC, Tosti A. A systematic approach to Afro-textured hair disorders: Dermatoscopy and when to biopsy. *Dermatol Clin.* 2014 Apr;32(2):145–51.

9 Hair weathering
Antonella Tosti

The environment causes damage to the hair shaft that cannot be repaired and is more evident in the distal part of long hair.

Patients with hair disorders, particularly androgenetic alopecia, are more susceptible to hair damage, because their hair shafts are thinner and more easily damaged by environmental agents. Ethnicity is also important: African hair is very fragile and easily broken by mechanical forces, while Asian hair is very likely to be damaged by chemical procedures.

Patients with damaged hair most often complain of hair shedding or of reduced hair growth and do not realize that their hair problems are due to hair breakage. Dermoscopy is very useful for showing patients the signs of hair weathering, which include trichorrhexis nodosa, trichoclasis, trichoschisis, trichoptilosis, and bubble hair.

TRICHORRHEXIS NODOSA

Box 9.1 Trichorrhexis Nodosa (Figures 9.1 through 9.7)

- Acquired hair shaft disorder.
- Most common sign of hair weathering.
- Hair shaft shows white knots and fractures.
- Dermoscopy: Brush-like hair fracturing.

Trichorrhexis nodosa is a very common sign of hair damage that mostly affects the distal part of long, damaged hairs.

At dermoscopy, the hair shafts shows multiple white areas that correspond to the sites of swelling and future fracturing. These are more numerous on the shafts that have been lightened by chemical treatment or sunlight exposure.

At higher magnification, the areas of breakage resemble thrust paintbrushes, as they appear as the ends of two brushes aligned in opposition. Fractured shafts appear as brush-like, widened stumps. Small broken fragments are also commonly seen.

Clips, rubber bands, and pins can cause trichorrhexis nodosa due to hairstyling. It is very common in women with androgenetic alopecia who wear their hair tied back in a bun or in a ponytail to cover the thinning of the top of the scalp.

Ceramic flat irons reach very high temperatures and often cause severe trichorrhexis nodosa, which is more evident on the superficial hair shafts.

Proximal trichorrhexis nodosa can be a consequence of intense scratching; dermoscopy shows broken shafts with multiple knots and scalp excoriations.

In women of African ancestry, trichorrhexis nodosa causes diffuse or patchy alopecia. Hair fragments obtained with the pull or tug test typically present knots and brush-like ends, makes diagnosis simple.

Severe trichorrhexis nodosa can cause localized or diffuse matting, which is usually precipitated by friction. This is seen after prolonged bed rest associated with increased hair shedding or piling of the hair during shampooing.

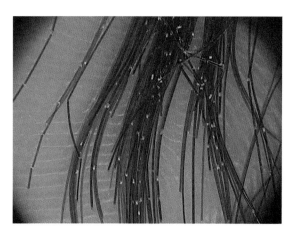

Figure 9.1 Trichorrhexis nodosa: multiple white areas along the hair shaft.

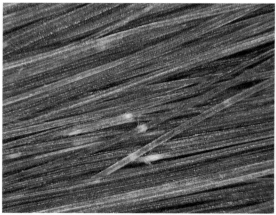

Figure 9.2 Trichorrhexis nodosa: multiple white areas along the hair shaft.

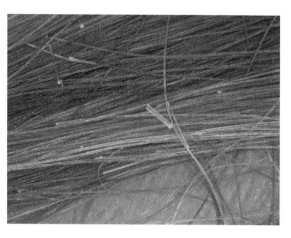

Figure 9.3 Trichorrhexis nodosa: note the presence of broken fragments.

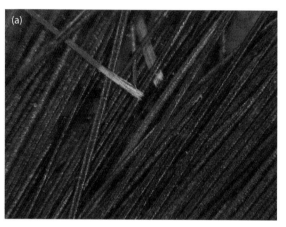

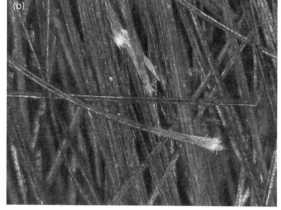

Figure 9.4 (a, b) Trichorrhexis nodosa: brush-like stumps.

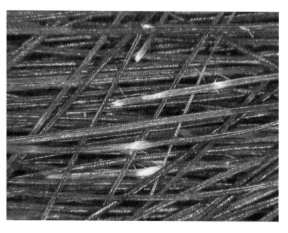

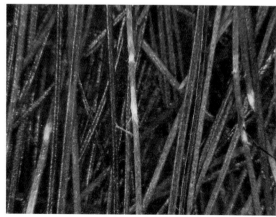

Figure 9.5 Trichorrhexis nodosa: the broken extremity resembles a paintbrush.

Figure 9.6 Trichorrhexis nodosa primarily affecting shafts that have been lightened by chemical treatment.

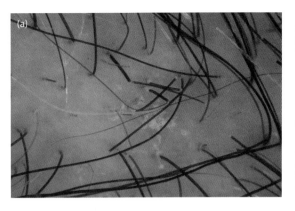
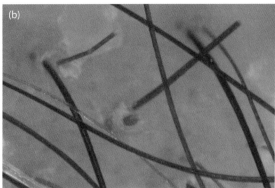

Figure 9.7 Proximal trichorrhexis nodosa due to scratching: note the multiple knots, broken hairs and scalp scaling (a). At high magnification, note the multiple knots (b).

TRICHOPTILOSIS (FIGURES 9.8 AND 9.9)

Trichoptilosis typically affects the tips of long hair that are split longitudinally into two or several divisions. The bifurcated hair shaft is typically not surrounded by cuticle. Central trichoptilosis is rare and almost exclusively seen in African hair.

Trichoptilosis is usually associated with other signs of hair damage, particularly trichorrhexis nodosa and trichonodosis.

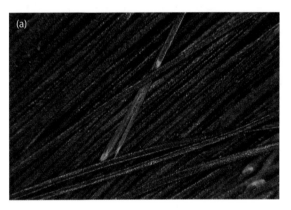
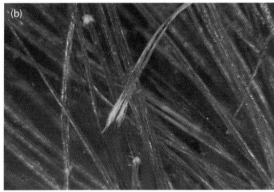

Figure 9.8 (a, b) Trichoptilosis: longitudinal splitting of the hair shaft. Note the thrust paintbrushes appearance of the tips.

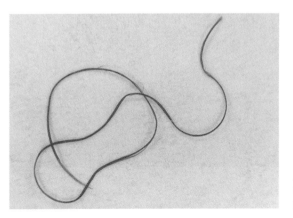

Figure 9.9 Central trichoptilosis in African hair. The central part of the shaft presents a fissure that does not reach the tip of the hair.

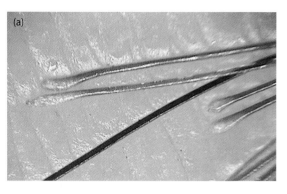
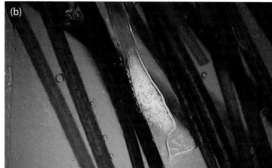

Figure 9.10 Bubble hair: the affected hairs have a white enlarged tip (a). Note the spongy appearance due to the presence of cavities at high magnification (b).

BUBBLE HAIR (FIGURE 9.10)

Bubble hair is due to the exposure of wet hair to very high temperatures from electric straighteners/curlers or blow dryers. This causes the sudden evaporation of water, with the formation of cavities filled with steam within the hair shaft. At dermoscopy, the affected shaft has a spongy "Swiss cheese" or "honeycomb-like" appearance due to the presence of bubbles of different sizes that distend the hair shaft.

TRICHONODOSIS (FIGURES 9.11 AND 9.12)

In hair knotting (trichonodosis), the hair shaft presents a single or double knot. The condition, which is more common in patients with curly hair, usually involves one or a few hair shafts and is caused by trauma due to friction, combing, brushing, and scratching. Hair knotting is very common in African hair.

Hair tangling and matting involves hair shafts with severe weathering. Dermoscopy shows trichorrhexis nodosa and raised cuticles.

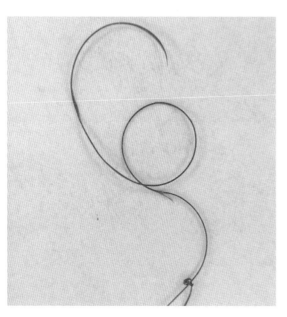

Figure 9.11 Hair knotting, trichorrhexis nodosa, and trichoptilosis in a fragment of African hair.

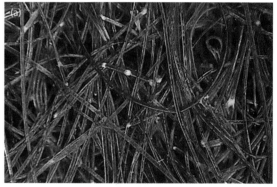
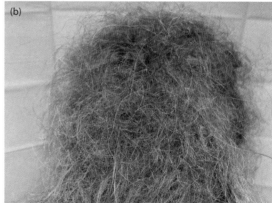

Figure 9.12 Severe trichorrhexis nodosa (a) in a patient with acute, irreversible matting (b).

EXTENSIONS (FIGURE 9.13)

Wearing extensions predisposes individuals to matting, as the telogen hairs that remain attached to the glued extensions easily tangle with the surrounding shafts. Clinical examination shows multiple white dots within the tangled area. These correspond to telogen roots entrapped by the glue at dermoscopy.

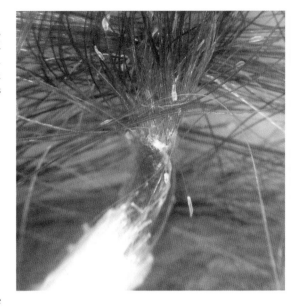

CAMOUFLAGE PRODUCTS (FIGURE 9.14)

Camouflage products are easily seen at dermoscopy: The most popular include fibers with electrostatic charges, powders, and crayons.

Figure 9.13 Numerous telogen roots are evident at the site of attachment of the extension.

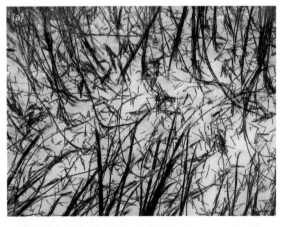

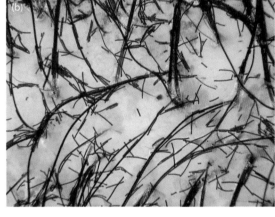

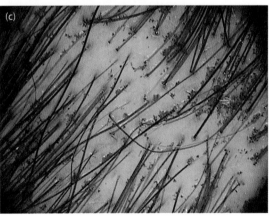

Figure 9.14 Presence of small pigmented fragments on the scalp surface (a). At high magnification, fragments have different lengths and are seen on the scalp and proximal hair shaft; also note the presence of hair dye on the scalp (b). Deposits of pigmented powder on the scalp surface (c).

HAIR COSMETICS (FIGURES 9.15 THROUGH 9.17)

Hair sprays can deposit on the hair shaft surface and irregularly coat the shaft at irregular interval. They are easily distinguished from true hair casts as their thicknesses and surfaces are irregular. Hair mousses can also leave residues on the shaft.

Permanent and semipermanent dyes can be detected on the scalp surface and within the follicular openings if the dye is not properly washed.

Keratin treatments: Patients can develop severe scalp irritation with scaling after keratin treatments. This is possibly due to contact dermatitis from formaldehyde, which is present or produced during the treatments. Dermoscopy shows severe scaling and arborizing and twisted vessels.

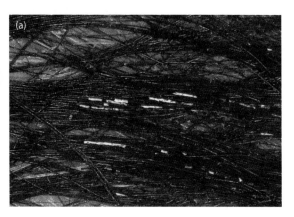 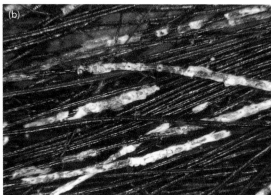

Figure 9.15 Hair spray deposits. White casts of different lengths surrounding the hair shafts (a). At higher magnification, the casts have irregular surfaces and thicknesses (b).

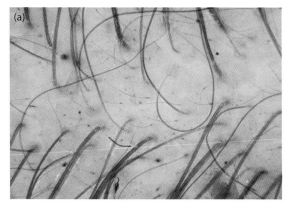 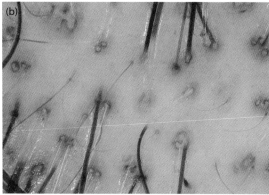

Figure 9.16 Pigmentation due to hair dye is present on the scalp surface and within the follicular openings (a). Hair dye penetration into the follicles is very evident at high magnification (b).

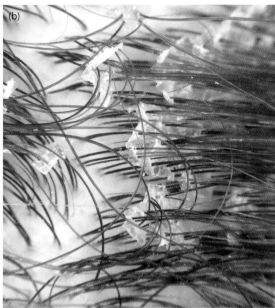

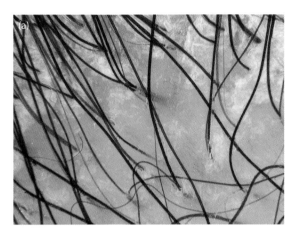

Figure 9.17 Scalp scaling with twisted vessels after keratin treatment (a). This patient experienced severe itching and shedding one week after the procedure; note the scaling around the proximal part of the shafts (b).

SUGGESTED READINGS

Miteva M, Tosti A. Dermatoscopy of hair shaft disorders. *J Am Acad Dermatol.* 2013 Mar;68(3):473–81.

Osorio F, Tosti A. Hair weathering, part 2: Clinical features, diagnosis, prevention, and treatment. *Cosm Dermatol.* 2011 Dec;24(12):255–9.

Rudnicka L, Rakowska A, Kerzeja M, Olszewska M. Hair shafts in trichoscopy: Clues for diagnosis of hair and scalp diseases. *Dermatol Clin.* 2013 Oct;31(4):695–708.

Yin NC, Tosti A. A systematic approach to Afro-textured hair disorders: Dermatoscopy and when to biopsy. *Dermatol Clin.* 2014 Apr;32(2):145–51.

10 Systemic diseases
Antonella Tosti

SYSTEMIC LUPUS ERYTHEMATOSUS

Box 10.1 Systemic Lupus Erythematosus (Figures 10.1 through 10.4)

- Acute telogen effluvium.
- Nonscarring patchy alopecia.
- Patchy alopecia due to discoid lupus.
- Dermoscopy: Enlarged branching vessels, short regrowing hairs, red dots and keratotic plugs.

Hair loss is a common complaint in patients with systemic lupus erythematosus, primarily during the disease's active phase. Patients may present with acute telogen effluvium, patchy nonscarring alopecia resembling alopecia areata or patchy scarring alopecia due to discoid scalp involvement.

Dermoscopy shows enlarged polymorphous vessels that are located interfollicularly or around the follicular openings (red dots). The patch shows short regrowing hairs and occasional keratotic plugs.

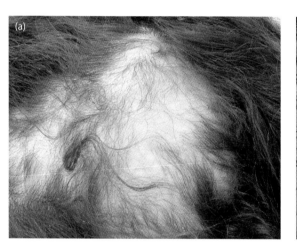 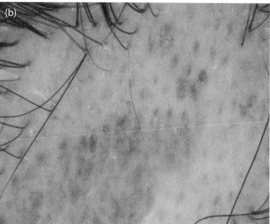

Figure 10.1 Systemic lupus erythematosus nonscarring patchy alopecia (a). Dermoscopy shows red dots and yellow dots (b).

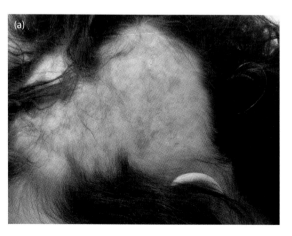 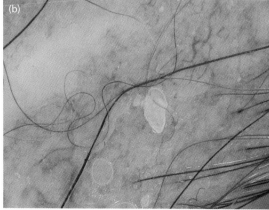

Figure 10.2 System lupus erythematosus scarring patchy alopecia due to scalp discoid lupus (a). Dermoscopy shows yellow scales and enlarged arborizing vessels (b).

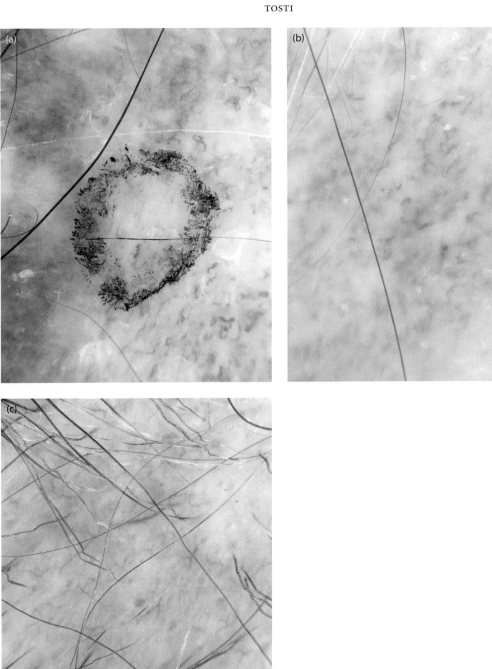

Figure 10.3 Polymorphous enlarged vessels within a patch of scarring alopecia (a, b). Also note the numerous pili torti (c).

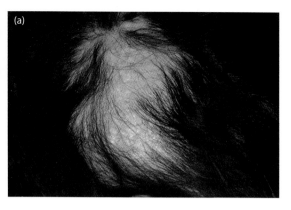

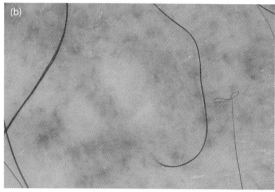

Figure 10.4 Dystrophic calcinosis cutis in a patient with scalp discoid lupus and systemic lupus (a). At dermoscopy, the calcific nodules appear as opaque white–yellow patches (b).

DERMATOMYOSITIS

Box 10.2 Dermatomyositis (Figure 10.5)

- Acute telogen effluvium
- Severe scalp itching
- Nonscarring diffuse alopecia
- Dermoscopy: Enlarged polymorphous interfollicular vessels

Nonscarring diffuse alopecia is common in dermatomyositis and is often associated with scalp erythema. Dermoscopy shows enlarged polymorphous interfollicular vessels.

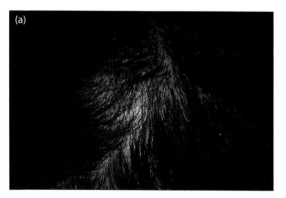

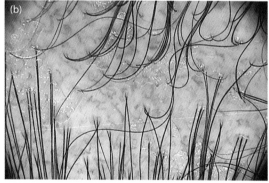

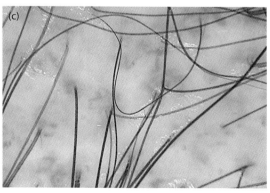

Figure 10.5 Dermatomyositis: diffuse alopecia with scalp erythema (a). Dermoscopy shows enlarged polymorphous interfollicular vessels (b, c).

SARCOIDOSIS

Scalp involvement from sarcoidosis is rare, but is most frequently reported in patients of African descent. Scalp sarcoidosis causes cicatricial alopecia due to the destruction of the hair follicles by the granulomatous formation. Early-stage disease presents with itching scalp papules and crusts. In longstanding cases, patients present with well-circumscribed patches of scarring alopecia with atrophic, erythematous, or yellowish skin.

Dermoscopy of early-stage disease shows normal or slightly reduced hair density and interfollicular and perifollicular yellowish-to-pale orange round spots, absence of follicular ostia and scaling. Established patches show a diffuse yellowish-to-pale orange discoloration, prominent telangiectasia, and few dystrophic hairs.

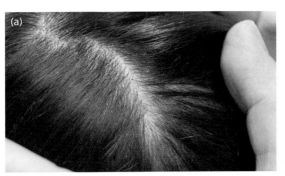
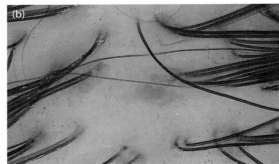

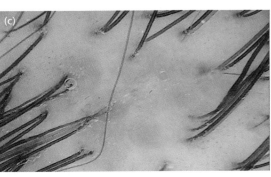

Figure 10.6 Early scalp involvement with papular and crusted lesions (a). Dermoscopy shows interfollicular and perifollicular yellowish-to-pale orange round spots with normal hair density (b) or within small areas with the absence of follicular openings (c).

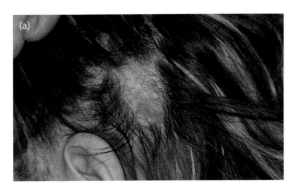
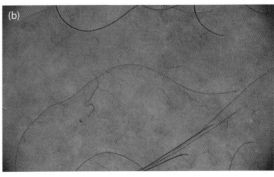

Figure 10.7 Well-demarcated patch of scarring alopecia. (a) Dermoscopy shows diffuse yellowish-to-pale orange discoloration with prominent telangiectasia (b) and a few dystrophic hairs at the patch periphery (c). *(Continued)*

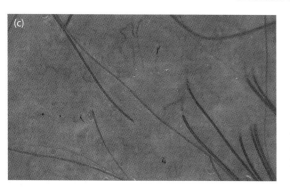

Figure 10.7 (Continued) Well-demarcated patch of scarring alopecia. (a) Dermoscopy shows diffuse yellowish-to-pale orange discoloration with prominent telangiectasia (b) and a few dystrophic hairs at the patch periphery (c).

CUTANEOUS T CELL LYMPHOMAS

Box 10.4 Cutaneous T Cell Lymphomas (Figures 10.8 and 10.9)

- Noninflammatory alopecia resembling alopecia areata
- Erythematous scaly patches of scarring alopecia
- Scalp nodular lesions with alopecia
- Dermoscopy: Diffuse erythema, scales, vellus hairs, black dots, and sparse broken hairs

Alopecia can be a feature of folliculotropic mycosis fungoides and of nonfolliculotropic cutaneous T cell lymphoma. It can affect the scalp or other hair-bearing body areas. Patients can present with noninflammatory patches of alopecia resembling alopecia areata or even alopecia totalis/universalis. In some cases, the alopecia is reversible. Other possible presentations include erythematous scaly patches of nonscarring alopecia and scalp nodular or ulcerative lesions with alopecia.

Dermoscopy can show features of nonscarring alopecia with vellus hairs, black dots, and sparse broken hairs or, in case of scarring patches, loss of follicular openings, dilated vessels, and scaling.

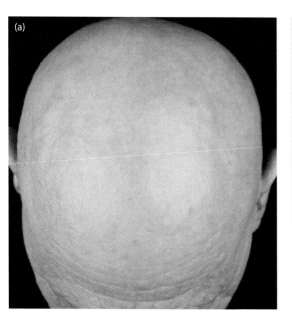

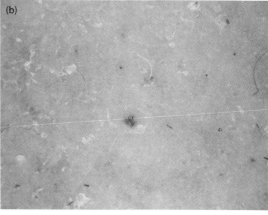

Figure 10.8 Cutaneous T cell lymphoma causing diffuse nonscarring alopecia resembling alopecia universalis (a). Dermoscopy shows features of nonscarring alopecia with broken hairs, black dots (b) and vellus hairs. (Courtesy of Dr. Laila El Shabrawi-Caelen, Graz, Austria.)

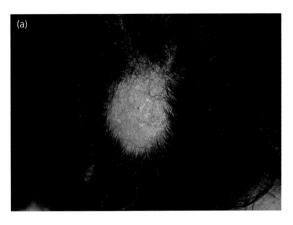
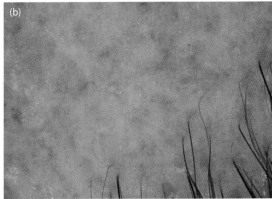

Figure 10.9 Folliculotropic mycosis fungoides. Patch of scarring alopecia with erythema and scaling (a). Dermoscopy shows loss of follicular openings, scales, and dilated vessels (b).

SYSTEMIC AMYLOIDOSIS

Box 10.5 Systemic Amyloidosis (Figure 10.10)

- Diffuse nonscarring alopecia
- Dermoscopy: Black dots and broken hairs surrounded by a yellow–pink halo

Alopecia in systemic amyloidosis is rare and presents as diffuse nonscarring alopecia. Dermoscopy shows yellow–pink halos surrounding the follicular openings. Broken hairs and black dots are also seen.

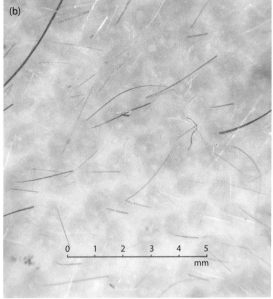
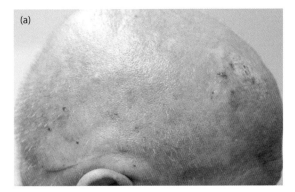

Figure 10.10 Systemic amyloidosis causing diffuse nonscarring alopecia (a). Dermoscopy shows reduced hair density and yellow–pink halos surrounding empty follicular openings and broken hairs (b).

SUGGESTED READINGS

Miteva M, El Shabrawi-Caelen L, Fink-Puches R, Beham-Schmid C, Romanelli P, Kerdel F, Tosti A. Alopecia universalis associated with cutaneous T cell lymphoma. *Dermatology*. 2014;229(2):65–9.

Torres F, Tosti A, Misciali C, Lorenzi S. Trichoscopy as a clue to the diagnosis of scalp sarcoidosis. *Int J Dermatol*. 2011 Mar;50(3):358–61.

11 Inflammatory scalp disorders
Colombina Vincenzi and Antonella Tosti

SCALP PSORIASIS

Box 11.1 Scalp Psoriasis (Figures 11.1 through 11.6)

- Psoriasis limited to the scalp is common and frequently misdiagnosed as seborrheic dermatitis.
- Dermoscopy helps diagnosis by showing typical vascular abnormalities.
- These are more visible in areas not covered by scales.
- At low magnification, vessels appear as red dots and globules.
- At high magnification (40× and more), multiple twisted capillary loops are seen both in the involved and apparently noninvolved scalp.
- Dermoscopic evaluation of the scalp can confirm the diagnosis of nail psoriasis or of atypical skin psoriasis.
- A photographic scale can be utilized for grading disease severity.

The scalp is the most commonly affected site in psoriasis (70%–80% of cases) and can often be the sole site of involvement. Psoriasis limited to the scalp causes scalp scaling and itching with a clinical picture that may closely resemble seborrheic dermatitis.

Scales can be silver white or yellow. In patients with oily skin, the scales usually have a greasy appearance (sebopsoriasis).

Hair loss is common, with a variety clinical presentations ranging from localized to generalized hair loss or even scarring alopecia.

Dermoscopy is very useful for confirming the diagnosis of scalp psoriasis. Dermoscopic features of scalp psoriasis are red dots and globules, twisted capillary loops, and glomerular vessels.

At low magnification (20×), the capillary abnormalities that characterize psoriasis are evident as an extensive array of red dots and globules. At higher magnifications, they appear as multiple interfollicular twisted capillary loops. This pattern is not limited to the scalp areas with evident scaling; it is also evident on the apparently noninvolved scalp. The number of twisted capillary loops correlates with disease severity.

Scalp examination is useful for confirming the diagnosis of psoriasis in patients with atypical skin lesions or nail lesions.

Scaling severity can be graded on a photographic scale, which can be utilized to evaluate the effects of treatments.

Dermoscopy is useful for the follow-up of scalp psoriasis as the number of twisted loops decreases in response to treatments.

The vascular pattern (red dots, globules, and twisted loops) can distinguish psoriasis from seborrheic dermatitis, in which dermoscopy shows arborizing vessels and atypical red vessels but not twisted loops.

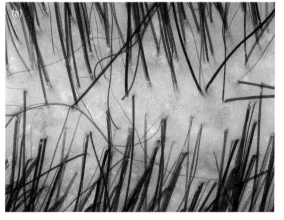
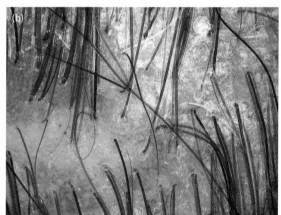

Figure 11.1 (a, b) Scalp psoriasis: red dots and globules.

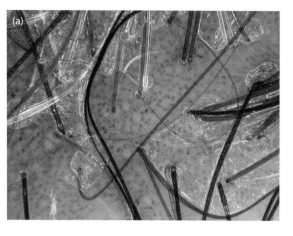
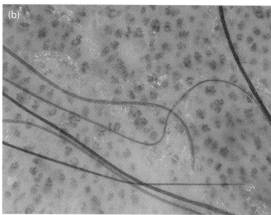

Figure 11.2 (a, b) Scalp psoriasis: twisted capillary loops.

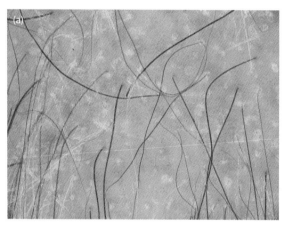
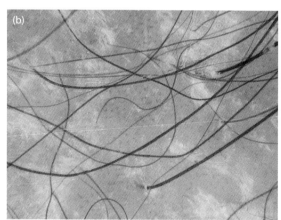
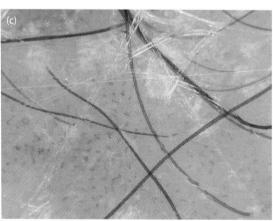

Figure 11.3 Scalp psoriasis: at low magnification, the scalp shows silvery-white scales and multiple red dots (a). At 40× magnification, the vessels appear as twisted loops (b); this pattern is more visible at 70× magnification (c).

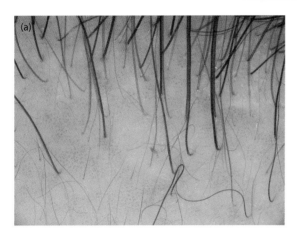
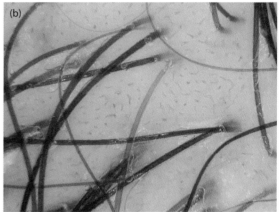

Figure 11.4 Scalp psoriasis associated with hair loss. At low magnification, the scalp shows multiple red dots, short regrowing hairs, and more than 20% hair shaft variability, indicating associated androgenetic alopecia (a). At high magnification, the twisted loops are evident (b).

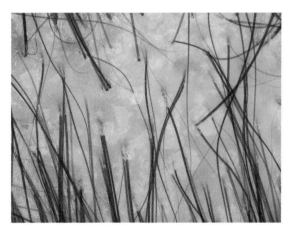

Figure 11.5 Sebopsoriasis: yellow greasy scales and red dots.

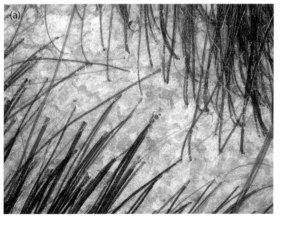
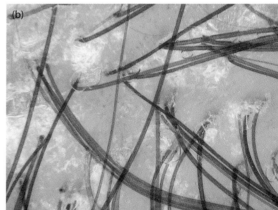

Figure 11.6 Scalp psoriasis: thick silvery scales do not allow for visualization of the vascular pattern (a), which can be identified in areas with less scaling at higher magnification (b).

SEBORRHEIC DERMATITIS

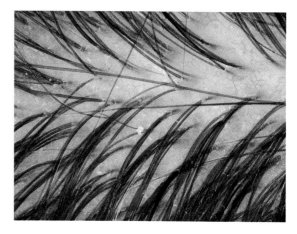

Figure 11.7 Seborrheic dermatitis: yellow greasy scales and arborizing vessels can be seen between scales.

Box 11.2 Seborrheic Dermatitis (Figures 11.7 and 11.8)

- Scalp involvement is very common.
- Erythema, scaling and, less commonly, small follicular pustules.
- Often associated with androgenetic alopecia and seborrhea.
- Dermoscopy: Yellow greasy scales and increased numbers of arborizing vessels.

Seborrheic dermatitis is a common scalp disorders in young adults that most frequently produces scalp scaling (dandruff) associated with mild erythema and itching.

The skin lesions often follow hairline recession in patients with androgenetic alopecia. Small follicular pustules and scalp excoriations can be observed.

Dermoscopy shows increased numbers of arborizing vessels, yellow greasy scales, small pustules, and excoriations.

CONTACT DERMATITIS

Box 11.3 Contact Dermatitis (Figures 11.9 and 11.10)

- Scalp lesions are uncommon, and patients usually complain of scalp itching.
- Erythema, mild scaling, and arborizing vessels are seen at dermoscopy.
- The dermoscopy pattern is not specific for diagnosis. In chronic cases, scratching induces a prominence of follicular ostia and proximal trichorrhexis nodosa.

Scalp contact dermatitis usually presents with severe scalp itching in the absence of typical eczematous lesions. Dermatitis of the ears, eyelid, forehead, or neck may be observed. Its most common causes are hair dyes, preservatives, fragrances, nickel, propylene glycol, and topical minoxidil.

Dermoscopy is not diagnostic but shows features similar to seborrheic dermatitis, including scaling and increased numbers of arborizing vessels. In chronic lichenified lesions, dermoscopy shows a prominence of follicular openings and proximal trichorrhexis nodosa due to scratching.

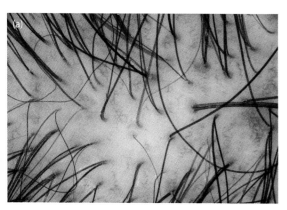
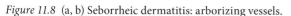
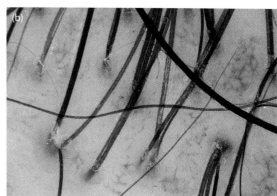

Figure 11.8 (a, b) Seborrheic dermatitis: arborizing vessels.

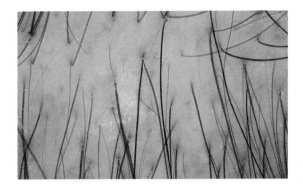

Figure 11.9 Scalp contact dermatitis: dermoscopy shows mild scaling and increased numbers of arborizing vessels.

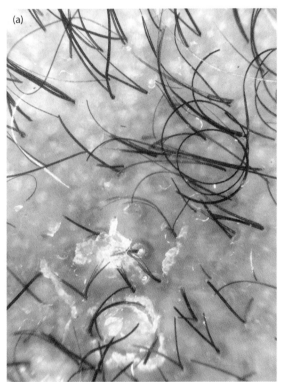

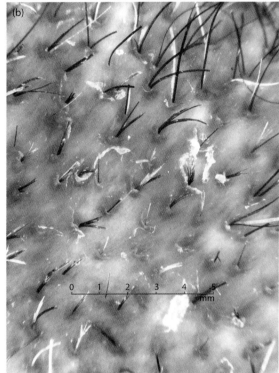

Figure 11.10 (a, b) Chronic scalp contact dermatitis: dermoscopy shows scalp scaling, prominent follicular openings, and proximal trichorrhexis nodosa.

SUGGESTED READINGS

Kim GW, Jung HJ, Ko HC, Kim MB, Lee WJ, Lee SJ, Kim DW, Kim BS. Dermoscopy can be useful in differentiating scalp psoriasis from seborrhoeic dermatitis. *Br J Dermatol.* 2011 Mar;164(3):652–6.

Ross EK, Vincenzi C, Tosti A. Videodermoscopy in the evaluation of hair and scalp disorders. *J Am Acad Dermatol.* 2006 Nov;55(5):799–806.

Tosti A, Donati A, Vincenzi C, Fabbrocini G. Videodermoscopy does not enhance diagnosis of scalp contact dermatitis due to topical minoxidil. *Int J Trichol.* 2009 Jul;1(2):134–7.

12 Infections
Antonella Tosti

TINEA CAPITIS

Box 12.1 Tinea Capitis (Figures 12.1 through 12.3)

- Common fungal infection, especially among children.
- Diagnosis is based on direct microscopic examinations and mycological cultures.
- Scalp scaling and alopecia due to hair breakage.
- Lymph node enlargement.
- Dermoscopy: Comma hairs, corkscrew hairs, black dots, broken hairs, hair casts, and transverse white bands.

Hair invasion by dermatophytes has a different epidemiology depending on the causative agent. *Trichophyton* species cause endothrix tinea capitis, which is the most common type in North America (*Trichophyton tonsurans*) and in Eastern and Southern Europe, and North Africa (*Trichophyton violaceum*). It affects both children and adults, transmission is interhuman and asymptomatic carriers are frequent.

Microsporum canis causes ectothrix tinea capitis, which is common in Western Europe and almost exclusively affects children. Transmission occurs through a symptomatic or asymptomatic animal, usually a cat.

Scalp scaling is a prominent feature in all types of tinea capitis. Tinea capitis produces patches of alopecia due to breakage of the hair shafts at the scalp level in endothrix infections or at 1–3 mm from scalp emergence in ectothrix infections. Pustular lesions may be observed in inflammatory tinea capitis (kerion). Cervical nodes are often enlarged.

The dermoscopic marker of tinea capitis is comma hairs, which appear as short C-shaped hairs due to bending of the hair shaft filled with fungi. Corkscrew hairs are seen in patients of African descent due to the shape of the broken hair shaft, which has a corkscrew or coiled appearance. Black dots, broken hairs, hair casts, and horizontal white bands ("Morse-code" hairs) may also be observed.

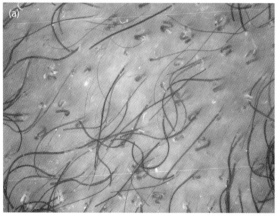

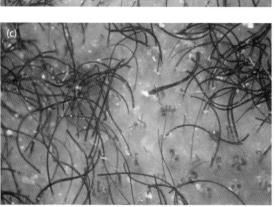

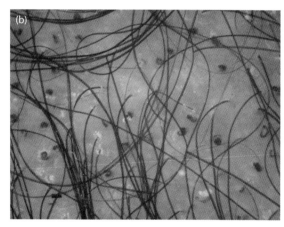

Figure 12.1 (a–c) Comma and corkscrew hairs in tinea capitis of patients of African descent.

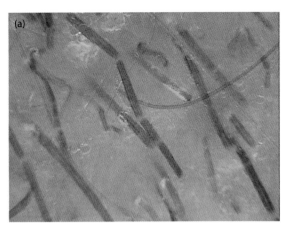
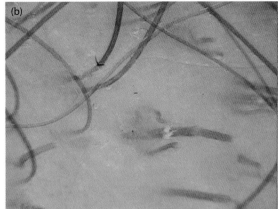

Figure 12.2 (a, b) Comma hairs and horizontal white bands.

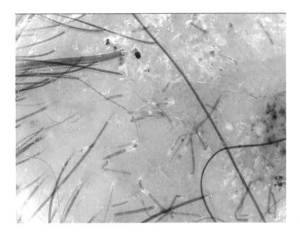

Figure 12.3 Comma hairs and hair casts.

PIEDRA

> *Box 12.2 Piedra* (Figures 12.4 through 12.6)
>
> - Superficial mycoses of the hair shaft that can cause hair breakage
> - White piedra: Yellow–white fusiform nodules
> - Black piedra: Irregular, dark, pebble-sized nodules
> - Dermoscopy: White or black concretions on the hair shaft

White piedra is caused by *Trichosporon asahii* and five other species of *Trichosporon*, a fungus that invades the hair shaft of pubic hairs, but it can involve the beard and scalp hair. The hair shaft is covered by soft yellow–white fusiform nodules, which are easily detachable.

Black piedra is caused by *Piedraia hortae*, a fungus that penetrates the cuticle, grows and then surrounds the hair shaft with hyphae. It mostly occurs in tropical regions and usually affects scalp hair. The clinical presentation consists of black, firmly attached, hard nodules on the scalp, beard, and body hair.

Dermoscopy shows white or black concretions on the hair shaft.

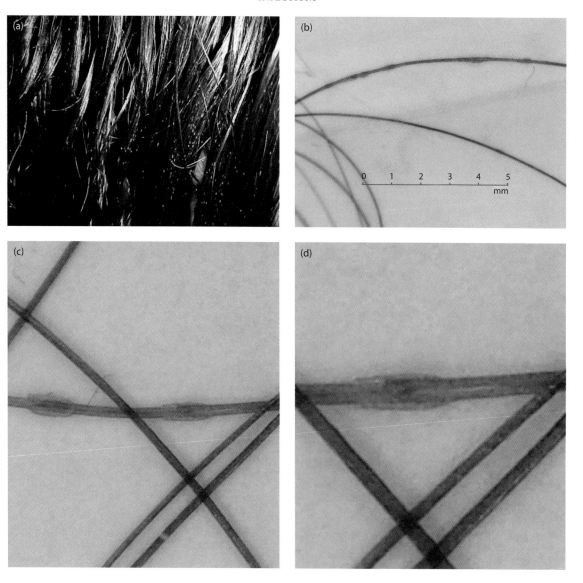

Figure 12.4 White piedra affecting the scalp of a Brazilian patient (a). (Courtesy of Dr. Nilton Di Chiacchio, Brazil.) Dermoscopy shows regular fusiform concretions surrounding the hair shaft (b–d). (Courtesy of Dr. Fernanda Torres, Brazil.)

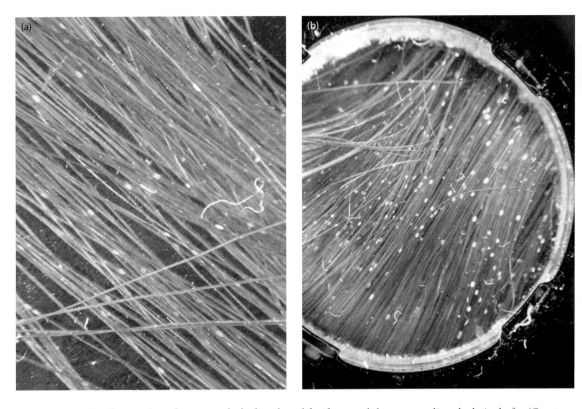

Figure 12.5 (a, b) White piedra: white, irregularly distributed fusiform nodules surrounding the hair shafts. (Courtesy of Dr. Lorena Dorado, Brazil.)

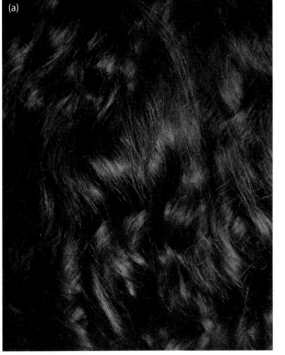

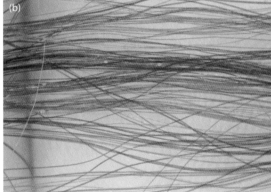

Figure 12.6 White piedra in a Brazilian woman with minimal clinical lesions (a). Diagnosis is confirmed by dermoscopy (b). (Courtesy of Dr. Leonardo Spagnol Abraham, Brazil.)

SUGGESTED READINGS

Haliasos EC, Kerner M, Jaimes-Lopez N, Rudnicka L, Zalaudek I, Malvehy J, Hofmann-Wellenhof R, Braun RP, Marghoob AA. Dermoscopy for the pediatric dermatologist part I: Dermoscopy of pediatric infectious and inflammatory skin lesions and hair disorders. *Pediatr Dermatol.* 2013 Mar–Apr;30(2):163–71.

Hughes R, Chiaverini C, Bahadoran P, Lacour JP. Corkscrew hair: A new dermoscopic sign for diagnosis of tinea capitis in black children. *Arch Dermatol.* 2011 Mar;147(3):355–6.

Khatu SS, Poojary SA, Nagpur NG. Nodules on the hair: A rare case of mixed piedra. *Int J Trichol.* 2013 Oct;5(4):220–3.

Pinheiro AM, Lobato LA, Varella TC. Dermoscopy findings in tinea capitis: Case report and literature review. *An Bras Dermatol.* 2012 Mar–Apr;87(2):313–4.

13 Parasitoses of the scalp

Giuseppe Micali, Francesco Lacarrubba, and Anna Elisa Verzì

PEDICULOSIS

- The diagnostic clues of pediculosis capitis (head lice) are represented by nits, which can be seen on close-up examination. However, they may be overlooked or misdiagnosed as scales of different origin or pseudo-nits (seborrheic dermatitis, debris, and/ or hair casts).
- In head lice, videodermatoscopy unequivocally shows the presence of nits, enabling a rapid differentiation from pseudo-nits and a more detailed identification of full versus empty nits.
- Videodermatoscopy may be also useful for the diagnosis of phthiriasis pubis (crab lice), which may occasionally affect the margin of the scalp and/or the eyelashes (phthiriasis palpebrarum).

Pediculosis capitis (head lice) is a worldwide parasitosis that is due to *Pediculus humanus var. capitis*, a bloodsucking insect and specific parasite of humans that predominantly affects children aged 4–14 years.

Generally, the diagnosis is clinical, as both mites and their nits are detectable upon close-up examination; however, searching for the mite is time-consuming and nits may sometimes be overlooked or misdiagnosed as scales of different origin or pseudo-nits (seborrheic dermatitis, debris, and/or hair casts).

Videodermatoscopy can be used as a diagnostic tool in head lice infestation, rapidly confirming the diagnosis in some puzzling cases in which parasites and nits may not be easily identified. It unequivocally shows the presence of lice (Figure 13.1) and full, viable nits (Figure 13.2), enabling a rapid differentiation from empty nits (Figure 13.3) and pseudo-nits (Figure 13.4), thus providing useful information regarding therapeutic responses [1,2]. Furthermore, videodermatoscopy does not require hair pulling, so a large scalp area can be investigated without discomfort to the patient. Moreover, videodermatoscopy enables an *in vivo* evaluation of the movements and physiology of lice, and may be useful for evaluating the pediculicidal activity of different topical products [3].

The same technique may be extended to phthiriasis pubis (crab lice), which is due to *Phthirus pubis* (Figure 13.5) and which may occasionally affect the margin of the scalp, especially in children, because of their lack of terminal hairs in other body regions. Moreover, videodermatoscopy may be useful in the diagnosis of phthiriasis palpebrarum [4], in which the crab lice are often difficult to identify because of their semitransparency and deep burrowing into the lid margin. In these cases, videodermatoscopy can rapidly reveal the presence of lice and/or nits (Figure 13.6a) and enable the clear differentiation from pseudo-nits (e.g. scales of atopic dermatitis) (Figure 13.6b).

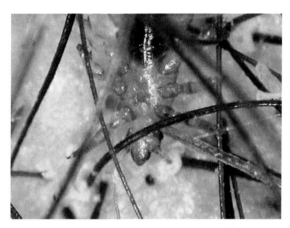

Figure 13.1 Videodermatoscopic observation (80×) of the scalp showing the presence of pediculosis capitis.

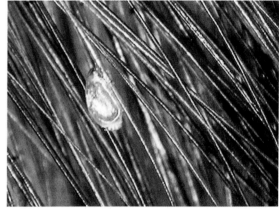

Figure 13.2 Videodermatoscopic observation (100×) of a full, viable nit.

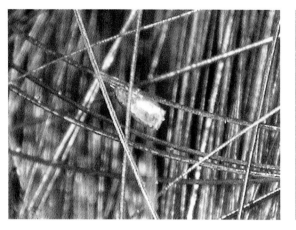

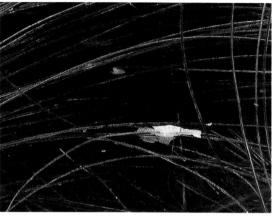

Figure 13.3 Videodermatoscopic observation (100×) of an empty nit.

Figure 13.4 Videodermatoscopic observation (100×) of a scale of seborrheic dermatitis.

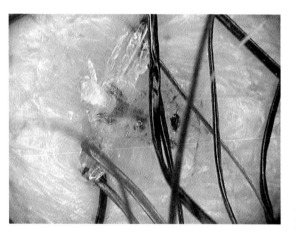

Figure 13.5 Videodermatoscopic observation (80×) of phthisis pubis on the skin.

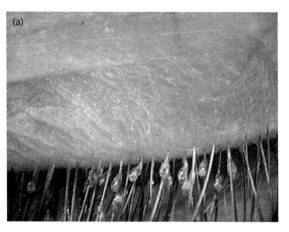

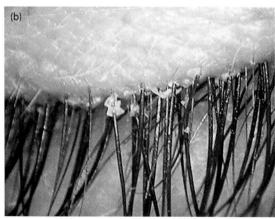

Figure 13.6 Videodermatoscopic observation (20×) of the eyelashes: nits in a case of phthiriasis palpebrarum (a) compared with scales of atopic dermatitis (b).

SCABIES

- Scalp localization of scabies is rare in adult immunocompetent patients, but might be responsible for cases of persistent infestation.
- Videodermatoscopy enables a detailed inspection of the scalp, with rapid and clear detection of the diagnostic signs of scabies infestation, such as burrows, mites, eggs, and/or feces.
- Videodermatoscopy is a simple technique for the diagnosis of scabies that can be easily used for routine observation of the scalp, especially in relapsing cases or in those who are resistant to therapy.

Scabies is a parasitic infestation due to *Sarcoptes scabiei var. hominis*. Scalp involvement is generally limited to newborn and immunocompromised patients showing the "Norwegian" or crusted form of the disease [5]. Scalp localization is rare in adult immunocompetent patients (Figure 13.7a–c), but might be responsible for some cases of persistent infestation due to the reservoir of the mite, as this site is generally spared from standard therapies [6,7].

Videodermatoscopy enables the detailed inspection of the skin, with the rapid and clear detection of the diagnostic features of scabies, such as burrows, at magnifications ranging from 40× to 200× (Figures 13.8 and 13.9), and mites (Figure 13.10), eggs or feces at higher magnifications (up to 600×). In most cases, an experienced observer is able to detect the mite moving inside the burrow. False-negative results are rare and there is no chance of false-positive results, as the images obtained are unequivocal. Videodermatoscopy is easy, rapid to perform, and well accepted by patients, as it does not cause physical or psychological discomfort. Moreover, it may be useful for the nontraumatic screening of family members and posttherapeutic follow-up [8–11].

In conclusion, videodermatoscopy is a useful noninvasive technique for the diagnosis of scabies. It can be easily used for the routine observation of the scalp, especially in those cases who are persistent or resistant to therapy.

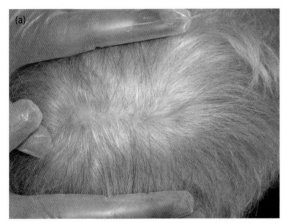
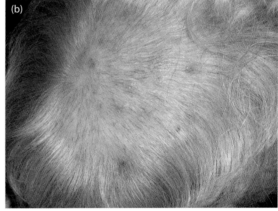
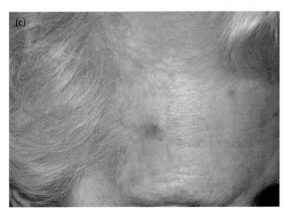

Figure 13.7 (a–c) Clinical images of a case of scabies of the scalp.

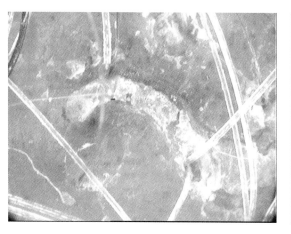

Figure 13.8 Videodermatoscopic observation (100×) of a burrow localized on the scalp.

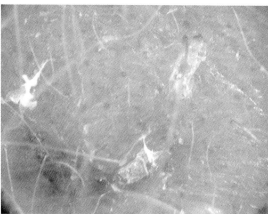

Figure 13.9 Videodermatoscopic observation (100×) of a forehead lesion, showing the presence of a burrow.

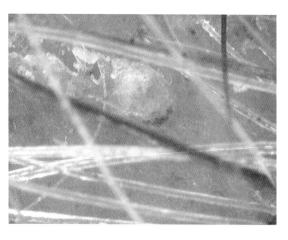

Figure 13.10 Videodermatoscopic observation (400×) of *Sarcoptes scabiei* localized on the scalp.

REFERENCES

1. Micali G, Lacarrubba F, Massimino D, Schwartz RA. Dermatoscopy: Alternative uses in daily clinical practice. *J Am Acad Dermatol*. 2011;64:1135–46.
2. Micali G, Tedeschi A, West DP, Dinotta F, Lacarrubba F. The use of videodermatoscopy to monitor treatment of scabies and pediculosis. *J Dermatolog Treat*. 2011;22:133–7.
3. Lacarrubba F, Nardone B, Milani M, Botta G, Micali G. Head lice: *Ex vivo* videodermatoscopy evaluation of the pediculocidal activity of two different topical products. *G Ital Dermatol Venereol*. 2006;141:233–5.
4. Lacarrubba F, Micali G. The not-so-naked eye: Phthiriasis palpebrarum. *Am J Med*. 2013;126:960–1.
5. Huang YC, Chen MJ, Shih PY. Photo quiz. Hyperkeratotic scales over the scalp. *Clin Infect Dis*. 2012;54:844–82.
6. Antonucci VA, Balestri R, Sgubbi P, Magnano M, Tengattini V, Bardazzi F. Atypical presentation of scabies: A single nodule of the scalp in a child. *G Ital Dermatol Venereol*. 2013;148:546–7.
7. Lacarrubba F, Micali G. Videodermatoscopy enhances the diagnostic capability in a case of scabies of the scalp. *G Ital Dermatol Venereol*. 2008;143:351–2.
8. Micali G, Lacarrubba F, Lo Guzzo G. Scraping versus videodermatoscopy for the diagnosis of scabies: A comparative study. *Acta Derm Venereol*. 2000;79:396.
9. Lacarrubba F, Musumeci ML, Caltabiano R, Impallomeni R, West DP, Micali G. High-magnification videodermatoscopy: A new noninvasive diagnostic tool for scabies in children. *Pediatr Dermatol*. 2001;18:439–41.
10. Lacarrubba F, Micali G. Videodermatoscopy and scabies. *J Pediatr*. 2013;163:1227–1227.e1.
11. Micali G, Lacarrubba F, Tedeschi A. Videodermatoscopy enhances the ability to monitor efficacy of scabies treatment and allows optimal timing of drug application. *J Eur Acad Dermatol*. 2004;18:153–4.

14   Body hair disorders

Antonella Tosti

KERATOSIS PILARIS

Box 14.1 Keratosis Pilaris (Figure 14.1)

- Keratinous plugs in the follicular orifices and varying degrees of perifollicular erythema.
- Extensor surfaces of the upper arms and legs.
- Associated with scarring alopecia in keratosis follicularis spinulosa decalvans.
- Dermoscopy: Single or tufted vellus hairs surrounded by peripilar casts. Coiled vellus hairs embedded in the horny layer.

Keratosis pilaris (KP) is a very common autosomal dominant disorder characterized by keratinous plugs in the follicular orifices and varying degrees of perifollicular erythema. It usually affects the extensor surfaces of the upper arms and legs.

KP is associated with scarring alopecia in keratosis follicularis spinulosa decalvans (KFSD), a rare X-linked or autosomal dominant disorder. Patients present with follicular hyperkeratosis, scarring alopecia of the scalp, eyebrows and eyelashes, corneal dystrophy, and photophobia.

Dermoscopy of KP shows vellus hairs surrounded by peripilar casts. Groups of two or three hairs may emerge together. In more severe cases, vellus hairs are coiled and embedded in the horny layer. Perifollicular erythema or hyperpigmentation is frequently seen. In KFSD, scalp dermoscopy shows a loss of follicular openings and peripilar casts surrounding single or tufted hairs (Figure 14.2).

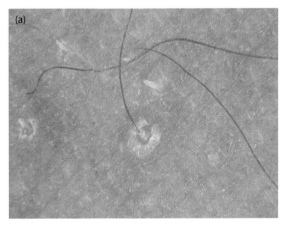 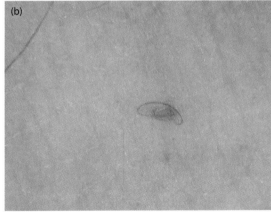

Figure 14.1 KP: peripilar casts surrounding vellus hairs (a) and coiled vellus hair embedded in the horny layer (b).

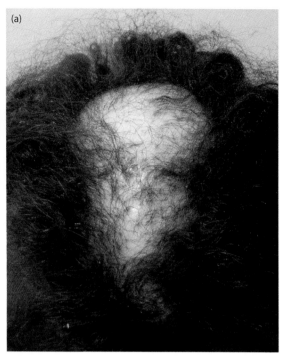

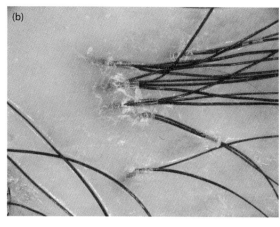

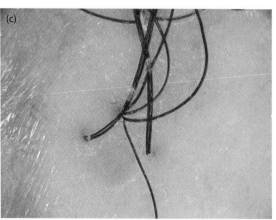

Figure 14.2 KFSD: scarring alopecia of the central scalp (a). Dermoscopy shows peripilar casts surrounding tufts of two or more hairs emerging together (b) and hair casts (c).

TRICHOSTASIS SPINULOSA

Box 14.2 Trichostasis Spinulosa (Figure 14.3)

- Retention of telogen vellus hairs within the follicle
- Itchy papulo-pustular eruption of the trunk and upper arms of young adults
- Comedo-like lesions of the face in the elderly
- Dermoscopy: Tufts of vellus hairs emerging from a dilated follicle

Trichostasis spinulosa is a relatively common disorder that results from the retention of 5 to 50 telogen vellus hairs within the follicle. It is most commonly observed in the face of the elderly, particularly on the nose, as comedo-like lesions, but can also affect young adults, where it produces an itching papular eruption of the trunk and upper arms.

Dermoscopy shows tufts of vellus hairs emerging from a dilated follicle.

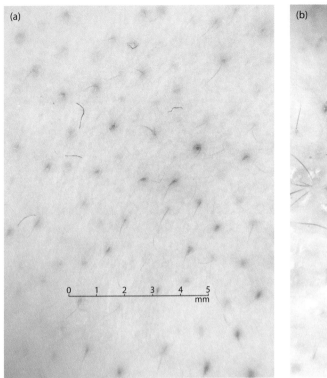

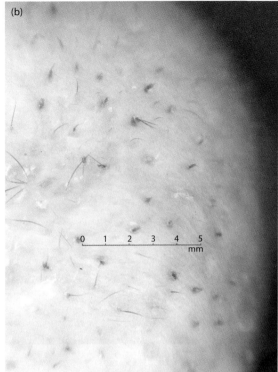

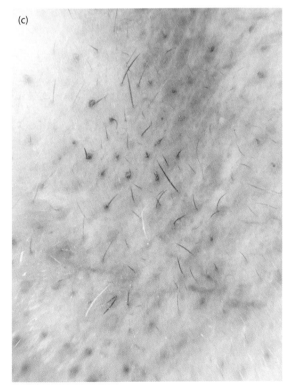

Figure 14.3 Trichostasis spinulosa: dermoscopy shows tufts of vellus hairs emerging from dilated openings (a, b) and yellow–brown follicular plugs (c). Also note the enlarged arborizing vessels due to associated rosacea.

CIRCLE HAIRS

Box 14.3 Circle Hairs (Figures 14.4 and 14.5)

- Dark hairs forming a perfect circle interspersed among normal hairs
- Overweight men with abundant body hair
- Abdomen, thighs, back, trunk, and upper legs
- Dermoscopy: Subcorneal hair coiling

Circle hairs appear as round, black circles interspersed between the normal hairs. The condition is asymptomatic and affects the abdomen, thighs, back, trunk, and upper legs of obese patients with abundant body hair. Circle hairs can occasionally be detected in the scalp.

Dermoscopy reveals perfectly circular (ring) hairs under a thin horny layer without follicular abnormalities or inflammation.

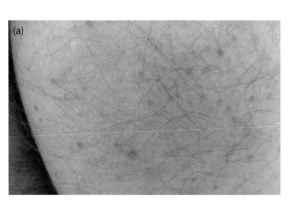

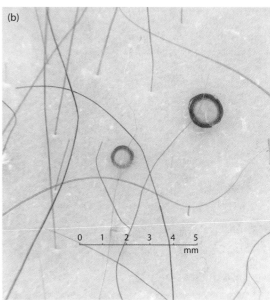

Figure 14.4 Circle hair: circle hairs are surrounded by normal hairs (a). Dermoscopy shows subcorneal hair coiling (b). (Courtesy of Dr. Martin Zaiac, USA.)

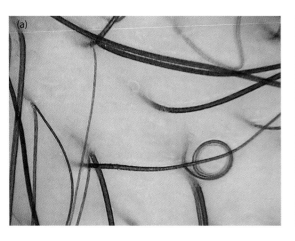

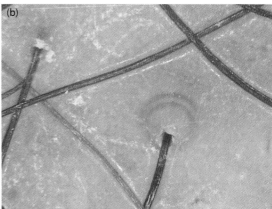

Figure 14.5 Circle hair: dermoscopy of a patient with androgenetic alopecia shows a subcorneal circle hair (a). A circle hair in the scalp of a patient with monilethrix (b).

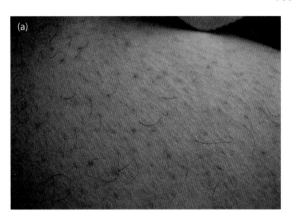
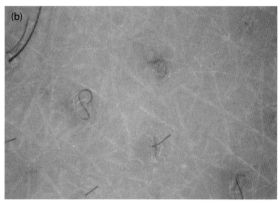

Figure 14.6 Rolled hair: inflammatory papular lesions with twisted hairs interspersed between normal hairs (a). Dermoscopy shows irregularly twisted subcorneal hairs (b).

ROLLED HAIRS

Box 14.4 Rolled Hairs (Figure 14.6)

- Possibly caused by mechanical traumas
- Keratotic inflammatory follicular lesions with twisted hairs
- Patients with other dermatological conditions
- Dermoscopy: Irregularly twisted subcorneal hair

Rolled hairs are more common than circle hairs and are possibly caused by traumas. Rolled hairs are usually seen in patients with other dermatological conditions applying topical medications. They present as keratotic inflammatory follicular papules with twisted hairs.

Dermoscopy shows irregularly twisted subcorneal hairs.

PSEUDOFOLLICULITIS

Box 14.5 Pseudofolliculitis (Figures 14.7 through 14.10)

- Papulo-pustular eruption mostly affecting the legs and groins or the beard and the nape area
- History of epilation with wax or plucking
- Hair shaft embedding with foreign body reaction and inflammation
- Dermoscopy: Hair shaft embedding

Pseudofolliculitis is common in women who depilate with techniques that produce ruptures of the shaft within the follicle (waxing, tweezing, and plucking).

The legs and groin areas show papulo-pustular lesions and pigmentary scars. Usually in this variety of pseudofolliculitis, embedding of the hair shaft occurs before its emergence (transfollicular penetration) from the skin and induces a foreign body reaction and inflammation.

Extrafollicular penetration is common on the necks of patients of African descent, where the hairs reenter the epidermis 1–2 mm away from their emergence.

Dermoscopy shows hair shaft embedding.

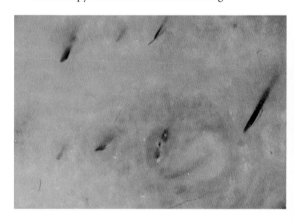

Figure 14.7 Pseudofolliculitis: dermoscopy shows embedding of the hair shaft before its emergence from the skin (transfollicular penetration).

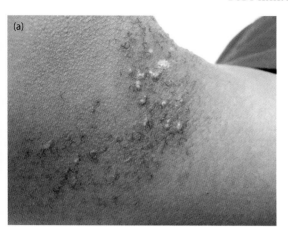
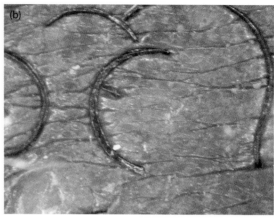

Figure 14.8 Pseudofolliculitis of the nape (a). Dermoscopy shows extrafollicular penetration. The hairs reenter the epidermis 1–2 mm away from their emergence (b).

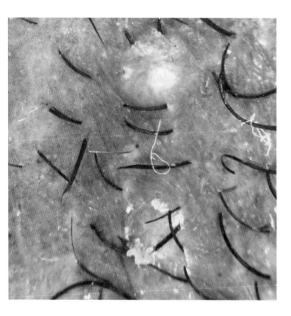

Figure 14.9 Pseudofolliculitis of the beard: dermoscopy shows extrafollicular penetration with pustules.

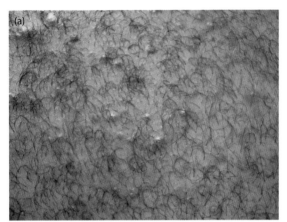

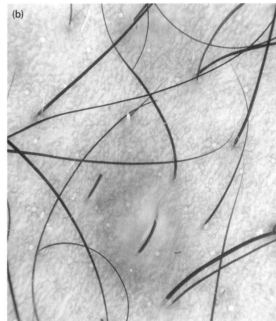

Figure 14.10 This patient developed pseudofolliculitis of the chest after waxing (a). Note the extrafollicular penetration (b).

SUGGESTED READINGS

Chuh A, Zawar V. Epiluminescence dermatoscopy enhanced patient compliance and achieved treatment success in pseudofolliculitis barbae. *Australas J Dermatol.* 2006;47(1):60–2.

Lacarrubba F, Misciali C, Gibilisco R, Micali G. Circle hairs: Clinical, trichoscopic and histopathologic findings. *Int J Trichol.* 2013;5(4):211–3.

Pozo L, Bowling J, Perrett CM, Bull R, Diaz-Cano SJ. Dermoscopy of trichostasis spinulosa. *Arch Dermatol.* 2008;144(8):1088.

Silverberg NB. A pilot trial of dermoscopy as a rapid assessment tool in pediatric dermatoses. *Cutis.* 2011;87(3):148–54.

15 Hair root evaluation
Antonella Tosti

PULL TEST

Box 15.1 Pull Test (Figures 15.1 through 15.4)

- Telogen roots
- Anagen roots without sheaths
- Anagen roots with sheaths
- Dystrophic roots
- Broken shafts

Dermoscopy allows for very fast evaluation of the hairs extracted via the pull test, which is an important step in the evaluation and diagnosis of patients with hair disorders.

Telogen roots are club-shaped and not pigmented. They are seen in the pull tests of normal subjects, as well as in the majority of hair disorders. Sometimes, telogen roots are surrounded by a keratinous envelope that encircles the proximal shaft; this indicates that telogen hair has been shed before the end of the telogen phase (premature teloptosis).

Anagen roots devoid of sheaths are typical of the loose anagen hair syndrome. They are pigmented and have a rectangular shape.

Anagen roots with thickened sheaths are typically seen in cicatricial alopecias and in pemphigus vulgaris.

Dystrophic anagen hair roots are hairs that are broken at the level of the keratogenous zone and present a fractured proximal end. They are typically seen in acute alopecia areata and in anagen effluvium. The shafts can also present irregular narrowing (Pohl–Pinkus marks).

In patients of African descent, the hair is fragile and breaks easily, and it is therefore very common to obtain broken hair fragments via the pull test. These should not be confused with dystrophic roots. Hair shafts also often show trichorrhexis nodosa and trichoptilosis.

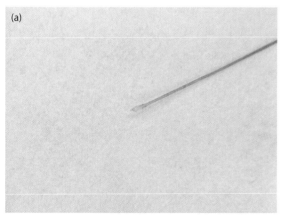

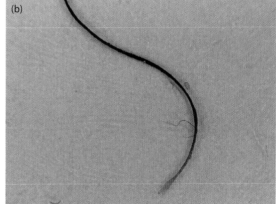

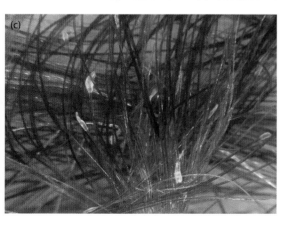

Figure 15.1 Telogen root: the root is club-shaped and not pigmented (a), even in cases of African hair (b). This picture taken of telogen hairs entrapped by extensions shows early telogen roots, which are characterized by the presence of a keratinous envelope (c); this is a sign of premature teloptosis.

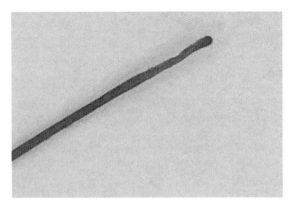

Figure 15.2 Anagen root devoid of sheaths in a patient with loose anagen hair syndrome.

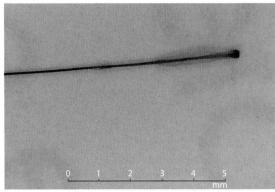

Figure 15.3 Anagen root with a sheath in a patient with lichen planopilaris. The root is pigmented and has a rectangular shape. The sheath is transparent and envelopes the proximal shaft.

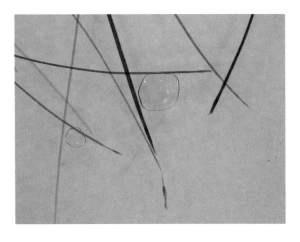

Figure 15.4 Dystrophic hairs in anagen effluvium.

TRICHOGRAM

Box 15.2 Trichogram (Figure 15.5)

- Confirms diagnosis of telogen effluvium
- Suggests diagnosis of androgenetic alopecia
- Diagnostic in loose anagen hair syndrome

Trichogram is a semi-invasive diagnostic test that is useful for assessing the degree of hair shedding and confirming diagnosis of telogen effluvium. The presence of thin short hair suggests associated androgenetic alopecia. It is the only test that can confirm diagnosis of loose anagen hair syndrome. Fernanda Torres recently described the "envelope trichogram," a method that utilizes the dermatoscope instead of the microscope to assess the type of roots in the trichogram. The plucked hairs are cut 5 cm from the roots and fixed with tape inside a transparent acetate envelope. The roots are then easily evaluated using the dermatoscope.

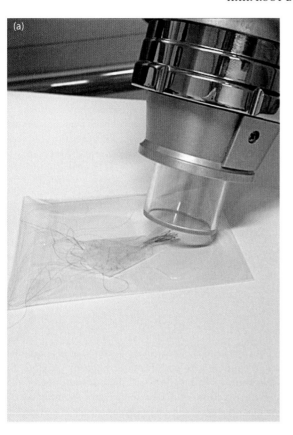

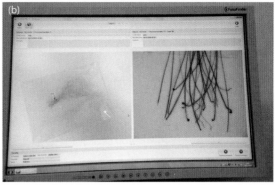

Figure 15.5 (a, b) Envelope trichogram.

16   Dermoscopy-guided biopsies

Antonella Tosti

Dermoscopy can be utilized to select optimal biopsy sites for pathological evaluation. This has been shown to increase the chances of a specific pathological diagnosis in cases of scarring alopecias, in which 95% of dermoscopy-guided biopsies yield a specific pathological diagnosis.

Dermoscopy-guided biopsies also enable the establishment of precise dermoscopic-pathological correlations.

Choosing which area to select depends on clinical suspicions and dermoscopic features. After selection, the area is marked, circled and a dermoscopic picture is taken.

HOW TO SELECT THE OPTIMAL SITE IN SCARRING ALOPECIAS

Box 16.1 Scarring Alopecias (Figures 16.1 through 16.5)

- Lichen planopilaris: Tufted hairs with peripilar casts
- Frontal fibrosing alopecia: Terminal hairs with peripilar casts
- Discoid lupus erythematosus: Keratotic plugs and red dots
- Folliculitis decalvans: Tufts of six or more hairs emerging together
- Central centrifugal cicatricial alopecia: White–gray halos and broken hairs

---

In lichen planopilaris and frontal fibrosing alopecia, disease activity is indicated by peripilar casts at dermoscopy. These may be very evident or subtle and difficult to distinguish from perifollicular scaling of seborrheic dermatitis. When changes are subtle, it is better to select a biopsy site with tufts of two or three hairs with peripilar casts.

In discoid lupus erythematosus, the biopsy should be taken from an area with keratotic plugs or red dots. In folliculitis decalvans, disease activity is indicated by the presence of tufts of six or more hairs surrounded by peripilar scales. In central centrifugal cicatricial alopecia, the biopsy should include a single hair or a couple of terminal hairs surrounded by white–gray halos.

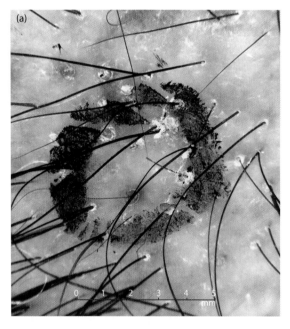
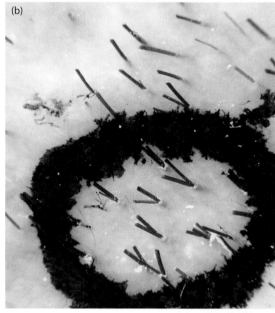

Figure 16.1 Lichen planopilaris: the biopsy site should include hairs with peripilar casts. These may be very evident (a, b) or subtle (c). When peripilar casts are not very evident, it is better to select a site in which the peripilar casts surround a tuft of two or more hairs emerging together (d).   *(Continued)*

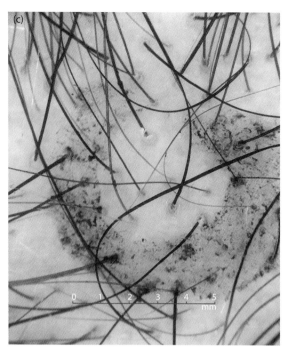

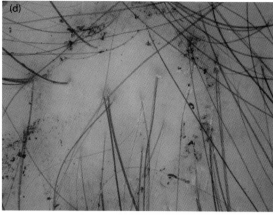

Figure 16.1 (Continued) Lichen planopilaris: the biopsy site should include hairs with peripilar casts. These may be very evident (a, b) or subtle (c). When peripilar casts are not very evident, it is better to select a site in which the peripilar casts surround a tuft of two or more hairs emerging together (d).

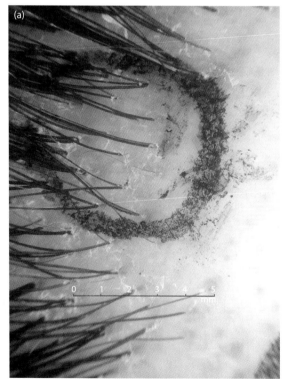

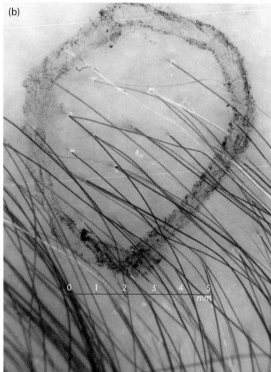

Figure 16.2 (a, b) Frontal fibrosing alopecia: the biopsy site should include terminal hairs with peripilar casts.

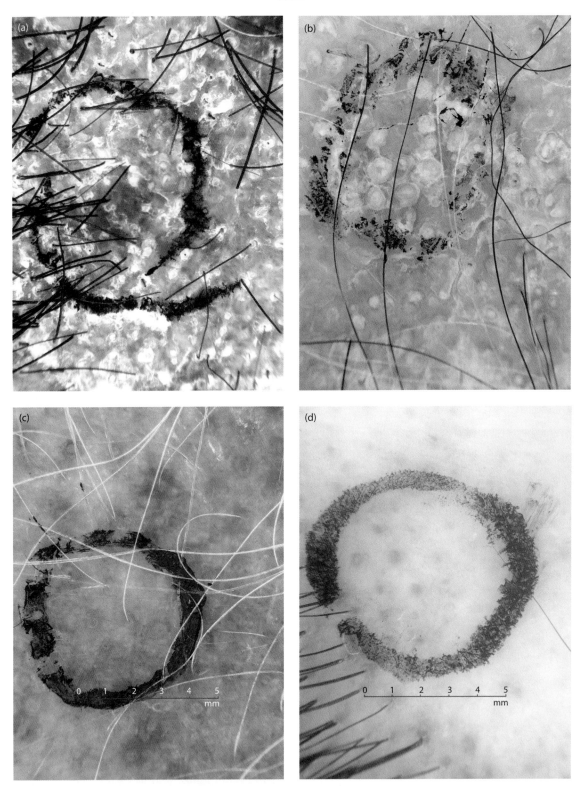

Figure 16.3 Discoid lupus erythematosus: the biopsy site is selected in an area with evident keratotic plugs (a–c) or red dots (d).

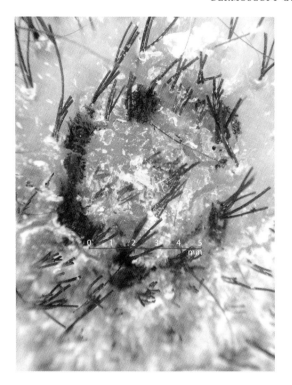

Figure 16.4 Folliculitis decalvans: the optimal biopsy site is selected in an area containing tufted hairs.

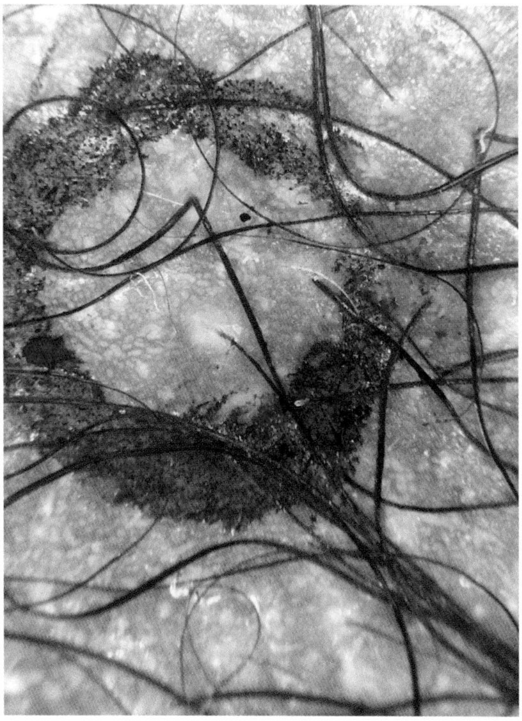

HOW TO SELECT THE OPTIMAL SITE IN NONSCARRING ALOPECIAS

Box 16.2 Nonscarring Alopecias (Figures 16.6 through 16.10)

- Alopecia areata: Exclamation mark hairs, black dots, broken hairs, yellow dots, and circle hairs
- Alopecia areata incognito: Yellow dots and short regrowing hairs
- Androgenetic alopecia: Hair diameter diversity
- Dissecting cellulitis: Yellow dots, broken hairs, and keratotic plugs
- Trichotillomania: Broken hairs and flame hairs

In alopecia areata, the optimal site should contain an exclamation mark hair. If this is not present, the biopsy site should contain black dots and broken hairs. In chronic alopecia areata, the biopsy site may be chosen in an area with yellow dots or circle hairs.

In alopecia areata incognito, the biopsy site should contain short regrowing hairs and possibly yellow dots.

In androgenetic alopecia, the biopsy should be taken from an area with hair diameter diversity and not on the vertex or in the area of parting in order to avoid a visible scar.

Figure 16.5 Central centrifugal cicatricial alopecia: the biopsy site is selected in an area with terminal hairs surrounded by white–gray halos.

In dissecting cellulitis, the biopsy should be taken from an area showing keratotic plugs, black dots, and broken hairs.

In trichotillomania, the biopsy site should include question mark hairs, if present, or broken hairs and flame hairs.

In traction alopecia, I prefer to select the site of biopsy at the margin of the patch in an area with hair casts.

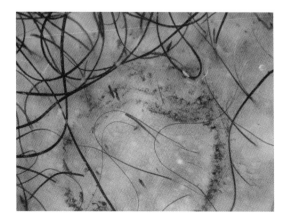

Figure 16.6 Alopecia areata: the biopsy site is selected in an area with broken hairs.

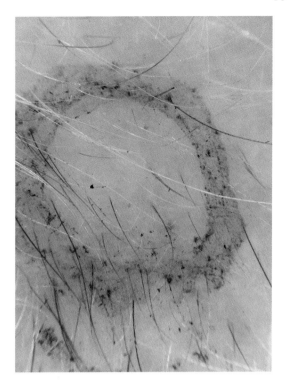

Figure 16.7 Alopecia areata incognito: the biopsy site contains short regrowing hairs.

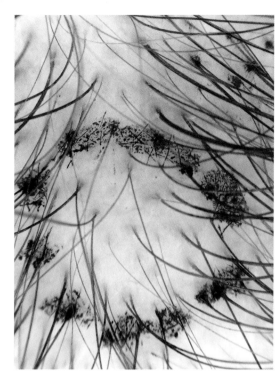

Figure 16.8 Androgenetic alopecia: the biopsy site shows hair diameter diversity.

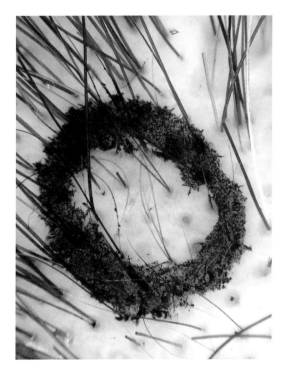

Figure 16.9 Dissecting cellulitis: the biopsy site contains a keratotic plug and broken hairs.

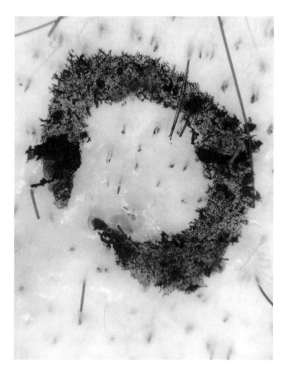

Figure 16.10 Trichotillomania: the biopsy site contains broken hairs and flame hairs.

SUGGESTED READING

Miteva M, Tosti A. Dermoscopy guided scalp biopsy in cicatricial alopecia. *J Eur Acad Dermatol Venereol.* 2013 Oct;27(10):1299–303.

17 *Ex vivo* dermoscopy
Antonella Tosti

Dermoscopy of biopsy specimen *ex vivo* can optimize the processing of horizontal scalp sections as it helps finding the correct level for bisection.

Specimens are laid horizontally over a piece of gauze and 20× magnification pictures are obtained with the dermatoscope lens pressed onto it. A transparent nonporous disposable plastic material (Parafilm®) is used to protect the lens of the dermatoscope from tissue contamination.

EX VIVO DERMOSCOPY OF SCALP BIOPSIES

Box 17.1 *Ex Vivo* Dermoscopy of Scalp Biopsies (Figures 17.1 and 17.2)

- Identify the dermoepidermal junction.
- The correct level of bisection is 1–1.5 mm below this line.

Contact polarized dermoscopy of scalp biopsy tissue enables the identification of the dermoepidermal junction in punch biopsy specimens. This appears as a clearly demarcated, brownish wavy line beneath the skin surface. The correct level of specimen bisection is 1–1.5 mm below the dermoepidermal junction.

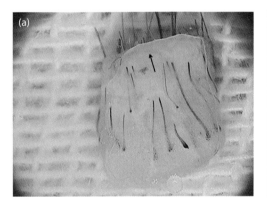 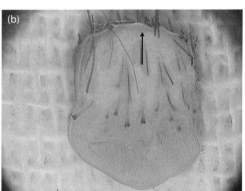

Figure 17.1 Ex vivo dermoscopy of a punch biopsy of androgenetic alopecia (a) and telogen effluvium (b). The dermoepidermal junction is marked with a black arrow.

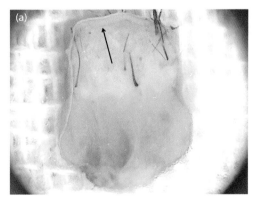 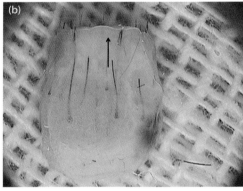

Figure 17.2 Ex vivo dermoscopy of a punch biopsy of lichen planopilaris (a), discoid lupus (b), and folliculitis decalvans (c). The dermoepidermal junction is marked with a black arrow. *(Continued)*

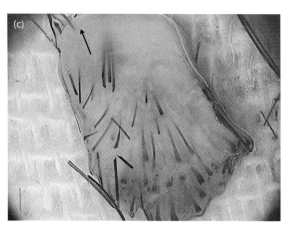

Figure 17.2 *(Continued)* *Ex vivo* dermoscopy of a punch biopsy of lichen planopilaris (a), discoid lupus (b), and folliculitis decalvans (c). The dermoepidermal junction is marked with a black arrow.

EX VIVO DERMOSCOPY OF SLIDES

The dermatoscope can be used to evaluate cut glass slides of horizontal sections. Pictures are taken against a white paper background using an iPhone®-attached dermatoscope, such as the Handyscope®. This enables emailing of the pictures from the laboratory to the pathologist in order to verify the size and orientation of the specimen.

Ex vivo dermoscopy enables the measurement of the size of the specimen. Specimens for scalp pathology should be of 4 mm, which is the size that allows for hair counts. It is also useful to evaluate whether the plane of the section is correct, so obliquely cut specimens can be reoriented. It also enables the evaluation of the level of the section (bulbar, isthmus, or infundibular).

> *Box 17.2* *Ex Vivo* Dermoscopy of Slides (Figure 17.3)
>
> - Measure specimen size
> - Establish whether the specimen needs to be reoriented
> - Evaluate the level of the section (bulbar, isthmus, or infundibular)

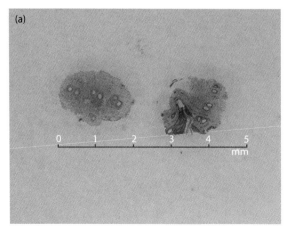

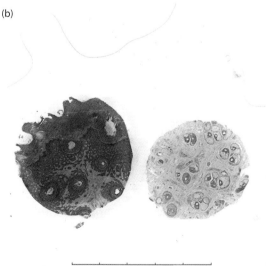

Figure 17.3 *Ex vivo* dermoscopy of a glass slide. The specimen size is too small and does not allow for a hair count (a). This specimen's size is correct, but the cut is oblique, so it should be reoriented for optimal evaluation (b). Size and orientation are correct (c). *(Continued)*

143

(c)

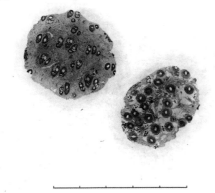

Figure 17.3 (Continued) Ex vivo dermoscopy of a glass slide. The specimen size is too small and does not allow for a hair count (a). This specimen's size is correct, but the cut is oblique, so it should be reoriented for optimal evaluation (b). Size and orientation are correct (c).

SUGGESTED READING

Miteva M, Lanuti E, Tosti A. *Ex vivo* dermatoscopy of scalp specimens and slides. *J Eur Acad Dermatol Venereol.* 2014 Sep;28(9):1214–8.

18 Dermoscopy in canine and feline alopecia
Fabia Scarampella and Giordana Zanna

DERMOSCOPIC FEATURES IN NORMAL DOGS AND CATS

> *Box 18.1* Dermoscopic Features in Normal Dogs and Cats (Figures 18.1 through 18.5)
>
> - Key differences between human and animal hair are in hair coat density and type of hair follicles.
> - Dermoscopy is very useful in order to better identify the characteristics of the normal hair coat of different breeds.
> - Dermoscopy may help with visualizing the normal blood vessel arrangements that are invisible under naked eye examination.

The skin formation in dogs and cats is quite different compared with humans based on histological findings such as hair follicles, epidermal thickness and layering, the presence of secretory glands, and epidermal cell proliferation.

In general, in animals, glabrous skin is present at the mucocutaneous junction, planum nasale and on the footpads, whereas the majority of the body surface is covered with hairs. An inverse relationship exists between the density of the hair coat and the thickness of the epidermis, with the hair coat usually being thickest over the dorsolateral aspects of the body and thinnest ventrally. Therefore, the epidermis is much thinner than in human skin, with one to three layers of living cells only in dogs, and slightly thinner than this in cats.

Dogs and cats have compound hair follicles with a characteristic spatial arrangement: groups of two to five primary hairs with a central, large, primary hair follicle are surrounded by five to twenty secondary hairs.

Both primary (outer-coat or guard hairs) and secondary (under-coat) hairs are medullated, and on the basis of their texture and length, they have been classified into different hair coats. For example, in dogs, three main classes of hair coats have been identified, and it is possible to better reveal the differences in their types by dermoscopy.

1. *Normal coat:* Composed of both coarse guard hairs and secondary fine hairs, with a high proportion of secondary hairs. This type of coat is typified by that seen in wolves or in breeds such as the German shepherd dog.
2. *Short coat:* May be coarse, as in Rottweiler or terrier dogs, with a strong growth of primary hairs and fewer secondary hairs than those in the normal coat. It may also be fine, as in dachshund or pinscher dogs, with the largest numbers of hairs per unit area and reduced primary hair size in comparison with the primary hairs of the normal coat.
3. *Long coat:* May be fine, as in chow chow or Pomeranian dogs, or wooly, as in poodles, with the highest number of secondary hairs (up to 80% of the total) in comparison with the normal coat.

In cats, differences also exist in the type of hairs. Recently, a dermoscopic study has revealed thick and straight hairs (guard hairs) emerging independently through individual external orifices in short-haired breed. All of these hairs were surrounded by three to four fine, slightly crimped, or undulating hairs (down hairs), all emerging through a common external orifice. Hairs that were thicker than down hairs but thinner than guard hairs were also detected and considered to be awn hairs.

All of these findings are different from those observed in long hair coat cats, such as Persians, which are characterized by a predominance of secondary hairs, or in partially molting breeds, such as Devon Rex, which is characterized by curly hairs with primary hairs that resemble secondary hairs.

In both dogs and cats, the blood supply to the skin is arranged into three distinct plexuses of arteries and veins lying parallel to the surface. By histology, it is possible to obtain a vertical view of blood vessels without the evaluation of their morphological features. By contrast, via a horizontal view of the skin, dermoscopy of the normal skin enables the identification of these blood vessels as thin arborizing vessels that are regularly distributed between follicular units.

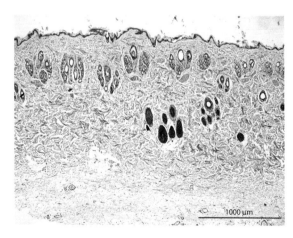

Figure 18.1 Normal haired skin of a cat. The epidermis ranges from one to two cell layers thick.

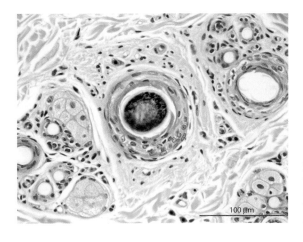

Figure 18.2 Transverse histological section of normal haired skin of a cat. Centrally, a large primary hair follicle is seen. The two compound hair follicles on each side of the central hair show a lateral primary hair follicle surrounded by three or four secondary hair follicles.

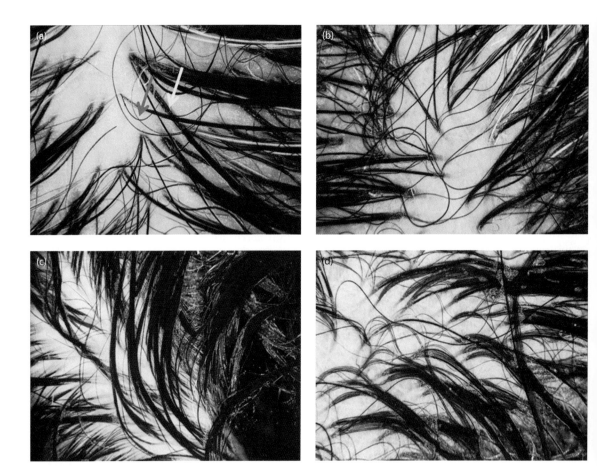

Figure 18.3 Dermoscopic features (70×) of hairs in different dog breeds, all from the lumbosacral region. Normal coat (a); primary hairs are indicated by the yellow arrow and secondary hairs by the blue arrow. Short coarse coat (b); note the predominance of primary hairs. Short fine coat (c); note the high number of hairs per unit area. Long wooly coat (d); note the high number of secondary hairs per unit area.

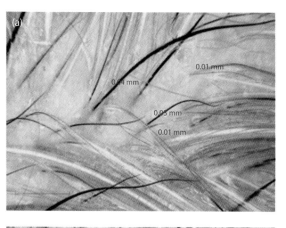

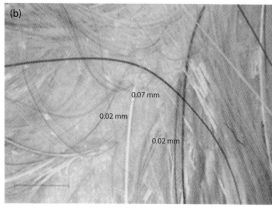

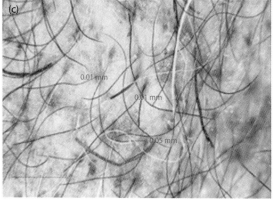

Figure 18.4 Dermoscopic features (70×) of hairs and their hair shaft thicknesses (scale bars: 1 mm) in different cat breeds, all from the lumbosacral region. Guard hairs appear as the thickest (0.04 mm) in comparison with awn hairs (0.03 mm) and down hairs (0.01 mm) (a). In Persian cats, secondary hairs are predominant on primary hairs (b). In Devon Rex cats, curly hairs are observed (c).

DERMOSCOPIC FEATURES IN SELECTED FOLLICULAR DISEASES

Alopecia and hypotrichosis are common clinical signs reported in several animal skin diseases. The most common causes of hair loss in dogs and cats are inflammatory alopecias.

FOLLICULITIS INDUCED BY INTRALUMINAL ORGANISMS

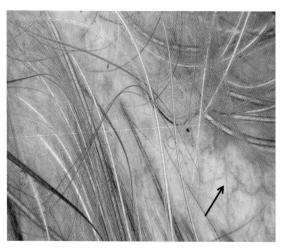

Figure 18.5 Dermoscopic features (70×) of blood vessels in the lumbosacral region of a dog. Thin arborizing vessels (black arrow) between follicular units are clearly observed.

Box 18.2 Folliculitis Induced by Intraluminal Organisms

- Most common cause of multifocal alopecia in dogs and cats.
- Dermoscopy is useful in the differential diagnosis of folliculitis induced by intraluminal organisms.
- Dermoscopy is useful for selecting the optimal specimens to confirm the diagnosis in folliculitis induced by infectious agents.

147

Folliculitis induced by intraluminal organisms is a type of alopecia in which an infectious agent evokes inflammatory cell invasion into the follicular lumen. This type of inflammatory alopecia mainly includes three infectious diseases in dogs and cats: demodicosis, dermatophytosis, and bacterial folliculitis. Dermoscopy may be useful in the differential diagnosis of some of these conditions and helpful for selecting the optimal specimens to confirm the diagnosis.

CANINE DEMODICOSIS

Box 18.3 Canine Demodicosis (Figures 18.6 through 18.9)

- Inflammatory alopecia common in young dogs caused by abnormal proliferation of *Demodex* mites within pilosebaceous units.
- Multifocal patches of alopecia, plugging, and variable amounts of scales and erythema on the head, legs, and trunk.
- Dermoscopy: Perifollicular scales, brown–yellow dots, peripilar casts, and follicular spikes.

Demodicosis is a common parasitic disease of young dogs characterized by the presence of a larger-than-normal number of *Demodex* mites within pilosebaceous units. *Demodex canis* is considered to be a normal resident of a dog's skin and it is supposed that the exaggerated proliferation of mites in young dogs is due to a genetic or immunologic disorder. By contrast, adult-onset demodicosis is a rare condition that, in most cases, develops due to an immunosuppressive disease or therapy.

Depending on the extent and severity of the lesions, two types of demodicosis are recognized: localized and generalized. The course of the localized form is benign and resolves spontaneously; by contrast, the generalized form usually covers large areas of the body and needs specific miticidal treatments.

Demodicosis usually presents as focal or multifocal patches of alopecia, erythema, and plugging on the head, legs, and trunk; in the generalized form, secondary pyoderma is often present, and in these cases, papules, pustules, and crusts are also observed.

Extensive and deep skin scraping demonstrating large numbers of mites is considered to be the most sensitive and specific diagnostic test for canine demodicosis. Trichography is a suitable and less invasive method, but requires a more careful selection of the sample sites.

The most common dermoscopic features observed at 10× magnification are reduced numbers of hairs per follicular unit, perifollicular scales, dilated follicular infundibula with brown–yellow keratotic material (brown–yellow dots), peripilar casts and the accumulation of keratinous debris, and sebum protruding from an empty follicular infundibulum (follicular spikes). Brown–yellow dots are more frequently observed in dogs with short hair coats.

Other dermoscopic findings include follicular micropustules (yellow areas), epidermal papillomatosis (in English bulldogs and pugs), and diffuse scales. No mites are clearly visible at this magnification.

Preliminary results of a study on dermoscopic–pathologic correlations in canine juvenile-onset demodicosis show that brown–yellow dots correspond to hair follicles, most of all those devoid of hairs, filled with keratin debris and *Demodex* mites.

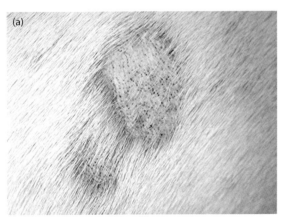
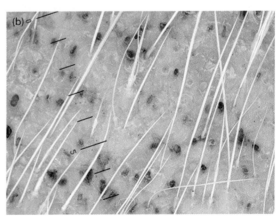

Figure 18.6 Clinical and dermoscopic features in two dogs with juvenile-onset demodicosis. Focal alopecia, papules, and follicular, plugging on the trunk of a French bulldog (a); in this case, dermoscopy at 10× magnification shows perifollicular scales and dilated follicular infundibula with brown–yellow keratotic material (brown–yellow dots) (b). Confluent areas of follicular plugging on the ventral aspect of the trunk of a shih tzu (c); in this case, dermoscopy shows accentuated follicular openings filled with keratotic material and peripilar casts (d). *(Continued)*

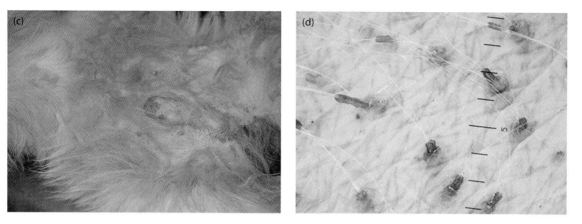

Figure 18.6 *(Continued)* Clinical and dermoscopic features in two dogs with juvenile-onset demodicosis. Focal alopecia, papules, and follicular plugging on the trunk of a French bulldog (a); in this case, dermoscopy at 10× magnification shows perifollicular scales and dilated follicular infundibula with brown–yellow keratotic material (brown–yellow dots) (b). Confluent areas of follicular plugging on the ventral aspect of the trunk of a shih tzu (c); in this case, dermoscopy shows accentuated follicular openings filled with keratotic material and peripilar casts (d).

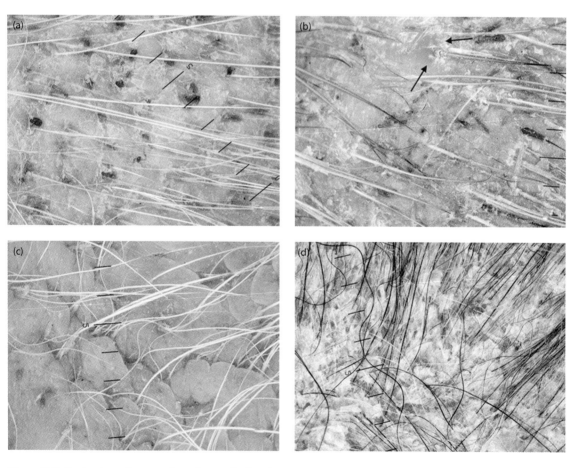

Figure 18.7 Canine juvenile-onset demodicosis: further dermoscopic features in different canine breeds. Brown dots and perifollicular scales in a pit-bull (a); perifollicular scales, peripilar casts, and follicular micropustules (arrows) in a French bulldog (b); epidermal papillomatosis and peripilar casts in an English bulldog (c); and diffuse scales in a Yorkshire terrier (d).

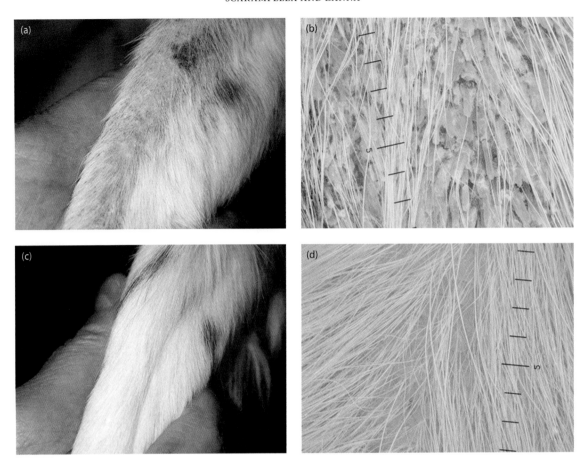

Figure 18.8 Canine juvenile-onset demodicosis: dermoscopy is useful for monitoring responses to treatment. Peripilar casts and the accumulation of keratinous debris and sebum protruding from several empty follicular infundibula (follicular spikes) as seen in a Cavalier King Charles with a very active disease (a, b). Peripilar casts and follicular spikes are no longer evident after three months of miticidal therapy (c, d) .

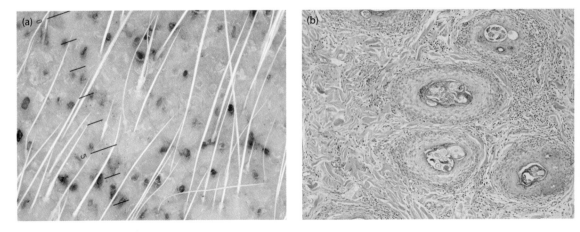

Figure 18.9 (a, b) Canine juvenile-onset demodicosis: dermoscopic-pathologic correlation. Brown–yellow dots correspond to follicles that are devoid of hairs and plugged with brown/yellowish keratotic material. Dermatopathology shows that the brown–yellow dots correspond to dilated follicular infundibula that contain keratosebaceous material and mites.

CANINE AND FELINE DERMATOPHYTOSIS

Box 18.4 Canine and Feline Dermatophytosis (Figures 18.10 and 18.11)

- Dermatophytosis is the most common pet-associated zoonotic disease and an early diagnosis is recommended in order to avoid the risk of contagion.
- Single or multiple patches of annular alopecia with scales, crusts and follicular papules, and seborrhea-like eruptions.
- Dermoscopy: Comma-like hairs and variable amounts of dry white-to-greasy yellow–brown scales.

Dermatophytosis is primarily a follicular disease and is the most frequent cause of inflammatory alopecia in cats. *Microsporum canis* is the most common cause of dermatophytosis in dogs and cats, but *Trichophyton mentagrophytes* and *Microsporum gypseum* infections have also been reported, particularly in dogs living in rural areas.

According to morphologic classification, two types of hair invasion are reported: endothrix and ectothrix. In endothrix infections, the hair shaft is filled by fungal hyphae, while in ectothrix, fungi produce masses of arthrospores on the surface of the hair in the keratogenous zone (Adamson fringe). In both cases, all hair shaft structures may be weakened.

The presence of ectoparasites such as fleas and *Cheyletiella* mites is suggested to be an important predisposing factor, especially in catteries. Genetic influences can also be important factors, as Persian cats and Yorkshire terrier dogs are more commonly affected.

Clinical signs of dermatophytosis in dogs and cats are essentially a reflection of hair shaft damage and subsequent inflammation. Single or multiple patches of alopecia with variable amounts of scales are the most common findings in both species. In cats, recurring chin folliculitis resembling feline acne and widespread papulocrustous dermatitis (miliary dermatitis) may occur. Subcutaneous nodules that are often ulcerated (dermatophytic pseudomycetomas) are seldom reported in Persian cats. In dogs, dermatophyte kerion, most commonly as a solitary lesion, may be observed on the face or a distal limb; these lesions are often associated with *M. gypseum* or *T. mentagrophytes* infections.

Methods utilized to confirm the diagnosis include Wood's lamp examination and direct microscopic examination of the infected hairs, but a definitive diagnosis is made via fungal culture or, in case of suspicious nodular lesions, via skin biopsy. These techniques have some disadvantages: only approximately 50% of *M. canis* infections are Wood's lamp positive, microscopic examination of plucked hairs may confirm the diagnosis in only 40%–70% of cases and the results of fungal culture may require weeks to be returned, leading to an increased risk of the contagion spreading between pets and between the pet and its owner.

In both dogs and cats, dermoscopy shows opaque, broken hairs characterized by a sharp slanting end and a homogeneous thickness, as well as variable amounts of dry white-to-greasy brown scales.

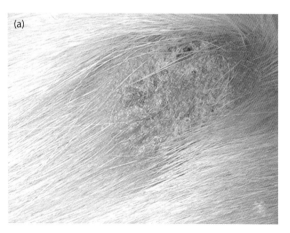
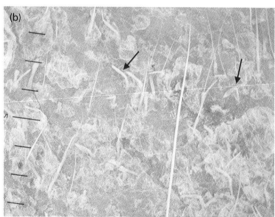

Figure 18.10 Canine dermatophytosis: clinical appearance of dermatophytosis in a Jack Russell terrier dog with *Microsporum canis*-induced dermatophytosis (a). Dermoscopy shows numerous broken, thickened hairs characterized by a sharp sloped end (comma-like structures) (arrows) and large, dry, white scales (b). In this case, dermoscopy was useful for monitoring response to treatment: hair grew back and comma-like structures were no longer evident after 20 days of antifungal therapy; instead, a few follicular plugs (brown dots) (arrows) and white scales were still visible (c, d). *(Continued)*

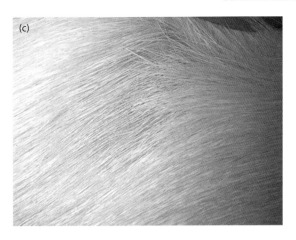 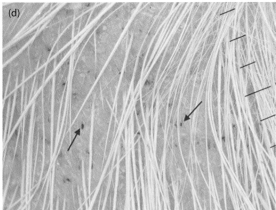

Figure 18.10 (Continued) Canine dermatophytosis: clinical appearance of dermatophytosis in a Jack Russell terrier dog with *Microsporum canis*-induced dermatophytosis (a). Dermoscopy shows numerous broken, thickened hairs characterized by a sharp sloped end (comma-like structures) (arrows) and large, dry, white scales (b). In this case, dermoscopy was useful for monitoring response to treatment: hair grew back and comma-like structures were no longer evident after 20 days of antifungal therapy; instead, a few follicular plugs (brown dots) (arrows) and white scales were still visible (c, d).

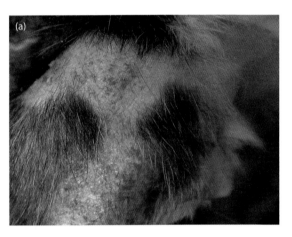 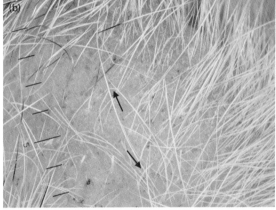

Figure 18.11 Feline dermatophytosis: clinical appearance of dermatophytosis on the ear of a European short-haired cat with *Microsporum canis*-induced dermatophytosis (a). At 10× magnification, opaque broken and thickened hairs with sharp sloped ends (arrows) are evident together with brown perifollicular scales (b).

CANINE SUPERFICIAL BACTERIAL FOLLICULITIS

Box 18.5 Canine Superficial Bacterial Folliculitis (Figures 18.12 through 18.14)

- The most common clinical presentation of pyoderma in dogs.
- Multifocal alopecia with follicular papules, pustules, and epidermal collarettes are the main presentations in short-haired dogs. In long-haired dogs, moderate-to-severe hypotrichosis, erythema, scales, and epidermal collarettes are observed.
- Dermoscopy: Yellow follicular pustules, yellow exudate, follicular casts, and perifollicular scales.

Canine superficial bacterial folliculitis is the most common cause of inflammatory alopecia in dogs, with *Staphylococcus pseudintermedius* being the most common bacterial agent involved. Because the condition is typically secondary to external or internal skin damage, the distribution of the lesions depends on the predisposing cause. The primary lesions are follicular papules and pustules that may be difficult to see in haired skin. In short-haired dogs, the initial clinical presentation in the involved areas includes small groups of hairs tufting together and rising above the skin surface. As the disease progresses, multifocal alopecia with or without follicular papules and scales, epidermal collarettes and hyperpigmentation become evident. In English bulldogs, multiple areas of alopecia and hyperkeratosis are reported as characteristic features.

In long-haired dogs, the initial clinical presentation may be only a loss of the luster of the hairs and mild hypotrichosis; with time, hair loss increases and erythema, scales and epidermal collarettes become evident.

The most common dermoscopic features observed at 10× magnification are reduced numbers of hairs per follicular unit, yellow follicular pustules, yellow exudate, follicular casts, and yellowish perifollicular scales. In English bulldogs and boxers, white-to-yellow diffuse scales are often seen.

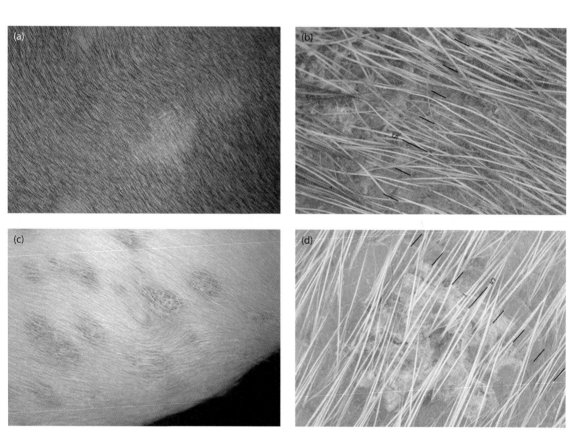

Figure 18.12 Canine superficial bacterial folliculitis in short-haired dogs. Initial clinical presentation: multifocal patches of alopecia on the trunk of a pit-bull (a). Dermoscopy shows erythema, scales, and a reduced number of hairs per follicular unit (b). Active disease in a pit-bull with multiple yellow crusts on the trunk (c); in this case, dermoscopy shows multiple confluent follicular pustules with dry exudate and scales (d).

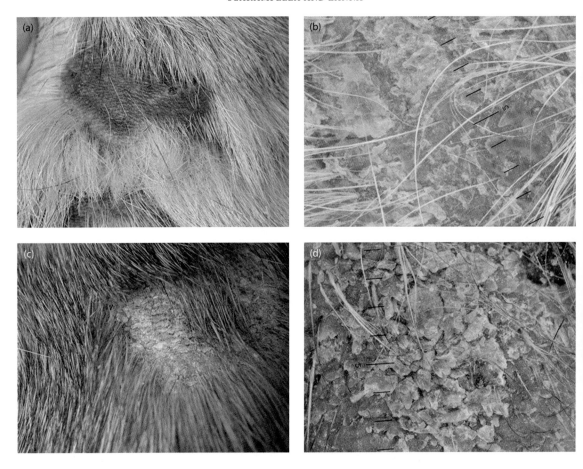

Figure 18.13 Canine superficial bacterial folliculitis in short-haired dogs: multiple patches of alopecia, hyperpigmentation, and collarettes in a pug (a); dermoscopy shows the presence of a dry yellow discharge on erythematous skin at the edge of the collarette (b). Focal alopecia with adherent scales in an English bulldog (c); dermoscopy shows a thick plaque of diffuse and follicular hyperkeratosis together with peripilar casts (d). These features are characteristic in this breed.

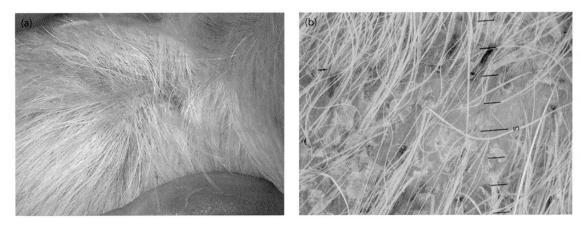

Figure 18.14 Canine superficial bacterial folliculitis in long-haired dogs: small crusts in a Maltese (a); perifollicular scales and tufts of hairs surrounded by yellowish peripilar casts are visible at 10× magnification in this case (b). Partial alopecia and scales in a long-haired mongrel dog (c); dermoscopy shows large scales and a dry purulent exudate (d).

(Continued)

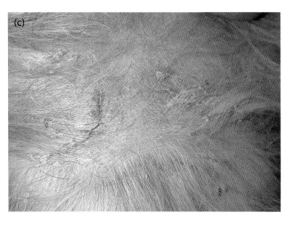

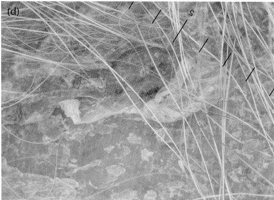

Figure 18.14 (Continued) Canine superficial bacterial folliculitis in long-haired dogs: small crusts in a Maltese (a); perifollicular scales and tufts of hairs surrounded by yellowish peripilar casts are visible at 10× magnification in this case (b). Partial alopecia and scales in a long-haired mongrel dog (c); dermoscopy shows large scales and a dry purulent exudate (d).

DERMOSCOPIC FEATURES IN NONINFLAMMATORY ALOPECIAS

Many noninflammatory alopecias in dogs and cats have long been described in various breeds. They are not all clinically uniform, but on the basis of their presentation, they have been classified into several disease entities.

CANINE PATTERN ALOPECIA

> *Box 18.6* Canine Pattern Alopecia (Figure 18.15)
>
> - Canine pattern alopecia is a relatively common but poorly defined skin disorder that affects different dog breeds.
> - Depending on the body areas involved, four syndromes have been recognized, all characterized by symmetric, progressive hair loss.
> - Dermoscopy: Hair shaft thickness heterogeneity, with a high number of thin hairs and a decreased number of hairs per follicular unit.

Canine pattern alopecia, which is also defined as canine pattern baldness, is a skin disorder similar to but is clearly not identical to androgenetic alopecia in humans. However, while in humans the genetic inheritance of this condition is well recognized, with a stepwise miniaturization of the hair follicle resulting in a progressive loss of hair diameter, length, and pigmentation, in dogs, the pathogenesis is currently unknown.

Two main syndromes are recognized in dogs:

- Pinnal-type pattern alopecia: Mainly described in smooth-haired and wire-haired dachshunds, it starts at approximately 6–9 months of age and

slowly progresses to involve the entire convex aspect of the pinnae at approximately 8–9 years of age. It is reported in both males and females, although males are more commonly affected.

Within this group, a well-recognized but poorly studied syndrome is represented by alopecia and melanoderma of the Yorkshire terrier. This is characterized by symmetric alopecia and marked, progressive hyperpigmentation restricted to the pinnae and over the bridge of the nose. It begins at 6 months to 3 years of age and affects dogs of either sex.

- Ventral-type pattern alopecia: Seen in several dog breeds with a short fine hair coat, such as dachshunds, Chihuahuas, miniature pinschers, whippets, or greyhounds, it starts at approximately 6 months of age and is characterized by a progressive alopecia developing on the base of the ear pinnae, ventral neck, the entire ventrum, and along the caudomedial aspect of the thighs. Hair loss is complete at approximately 1 year of age, remaining restricted to the aforementioned regions. It is reported in both males and females, although it is more frequently observed in females.

Within this group, a poorly defined disorder characterized by hair loss at the caudolateral aspect of thighs is seen in greyhounds. Although attempts have been made in order to detect an endocrine basis, no such results have been obtained.

Histologically, pattern baldness is characterized by a small diameter of hair shafts, with follicles being both moderately shorter and thinner than normal overall.

Although the diagnosis is usually based on clinical evaluation, the most common dermoscopic features observed are fine hair shafts (miniaturized) with a decreased numbers of hairs per follicular unit.

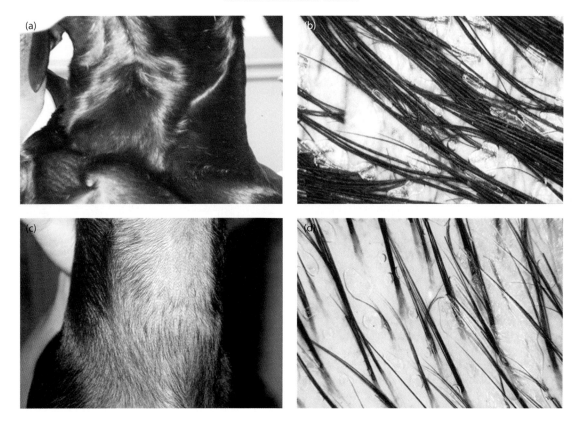

Figure 18.15 Clinical and dermoscopic features in a healthy miniature pinscher dog (a, b) and in a dog of the same breed affected by the ventral-type pattern alopecia (c, d). The images show the ventral neck region.

FELINE SELF-INDUCED ALOPECIA

> *Box 18.7* Feline Self-Induced Alopecia (Figures 18.16 and 18.17)
>
> - Acquired noninflammatory alopecia due to over-grooming.
> - Clinical features: Ubiquitous hair loss, mainly of a symmetrical distribution and often without other skin lesions.
> - Dermoscopy: Normal hair shafts suddenly and cleanly broken, hook-like and coiled hairs, oblique fractured hairs, and brush-like hairs.

Self-inflicted hair loss is a feline acquired noninflammatory alopecia due to over-grooming that may be associated with pruritic skin conditions or psychogenic disorders.

The main clinical sign of this condition is alopecia mainly in a symmetrical distribution on the abdomen, groin, lumbar and flank regions and on the lateral surfaces of the hind-limbs.

In some cases, there may also be evidence of papulocrustous dermatitis (miliary dermatitis) or secondary excoriations and a generalized increase in skin scaling.

Microscopic examination of broken hairs enables the distinguishing of self-induced from spontaneous alopecia.

Dermoscopy of self-induced alopecia shows normal hair shafts that are suddenly and cleanly broken at different lengths, suggesting a mechanical trauma. Other peculiar findings are hook-like and coiled hairs, oblique fractured hairs, and short tufts of hairs broken at equal levels and emerging from the same follicular opening. These features are possibly formed by hair pulling and, in the case of short tufts of hairs, by hair chewing. Brown dots and follicular casts are also observed in Persian cats.

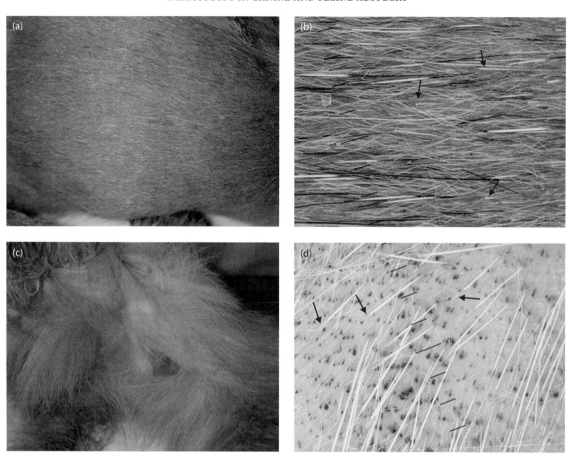

Figure 18.16 Feline self-induced alopecia: diffuse alopecia on the right flank of a domestic short-haired cat (a); dermoscopy shows normal hair shafts that are suddenly and cleanly broken at different lengths (arrows), (b). Feline self-induced alopecia in a Persian cat (c); broken hairs, oblique fractured hairs (arrows), and brown dots are shown (d).

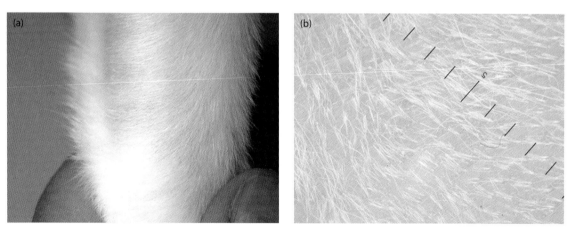

Figure 18.17 Feline self-induced alopecia: focal alopecia on the forearm of an allergic cat (a); at 10× magnification, short tufts of hairs broken at equal levels and emerging from the same follicular opening are visible (b). Multifocal alopecia on the ears of an allergic cat (c); dermoscopy shows areas of complete alopecia, scales, peripilar casts, and hook-like hairs (arrows) (d).   (*Continued*)

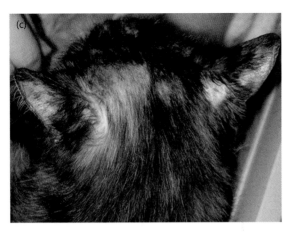
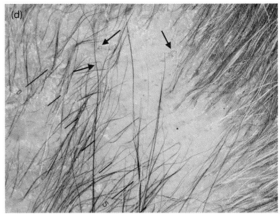

Figure 18.17 (Continued) Feline self-induced alopecia: focal alopecia on the forearm of an allergic cat (a); at 10× magnification, short tufts of hairs broken at equal levels and emerging from the same follicular opening are visible (b). Multifocal alopecia on the ears of an allergic cat (c); dermoscopy shows areas of complete alopecia, scales, peripilar casts, and hook-like hairs (arrows) (d).

SUGGESTED READINGS

Mecklenburg L, Linek M, Tobin DJ, eds. *Hair Loss Disorders in Domestic Animals.* 1st edition. Wiley-Blackwell, Ames, IA, 2009.

Miller WH, Griffin CE, Campbell KL, eds. *Muller and Kirk's Small Animal Dermatology.* 7th edition. Elsevier, St. Louis, MO, 2013.

Zanna G, Auriemma E, Arrighi S, Attanasi A, Zini E, Scarampella F. Dermoscopic evaluation of skin in healthy cats. *Vet Derm.* 2014; doi: 10.111/vde.12179.

19 Dermoscopy of the nail plate

Antonella Tosti

Nonpolarized dermoscopy of the nail plate requires the use of a gel (ultrasound gel or cosmetic gel) due to the convex shape of the nail plate. This gel fills the gap between the convex nail surface and the handheld or videodermoscopy device. Polarized dermoscopy without an interface solution can also be utilized with good results.

Box 19.1 Nail Plate Dermoscopy (Figures 19.1 through 19.5)

- Nail pigmentation
- Nail plate surface abnormalities
- Onychomycosis
- Traumatic onycholysis
- Psoriasis
- Other inflammatory nail disorders
- Nonpigmented tumors

Nail plate dermoscopy has been mainly utilized for the evaluation of nail pigmentation.

The diagnosis and follow-up of other nail diseases can also possibly benefit from the use of dermoscopy, as it may detect subclinical nail plate surface abnormalities, visualize the progression of onychomycosis, show abnormalities in the nail bed vessels and possibly be helpful in the diagnosis of nonpigmented tumors of the nail.

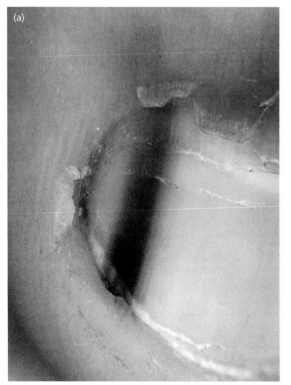

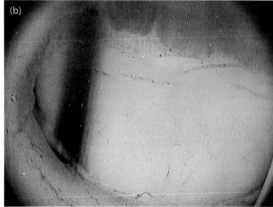

Figure 19.1 Nail plate dermoscopy in melanonychia: longitudinal melanonychia in a black child. Pictures taken with nonpolarized (a) and polarized dermoscopy (b) show a dark black band—pseudo-Hutchinson's sign. Pathology showed a nail matrix nevus.

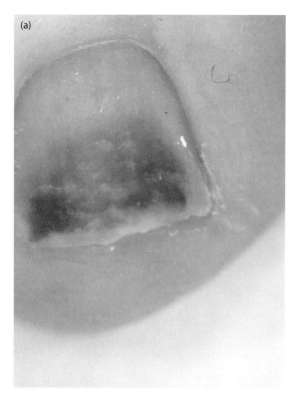

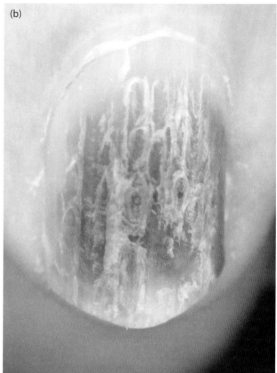

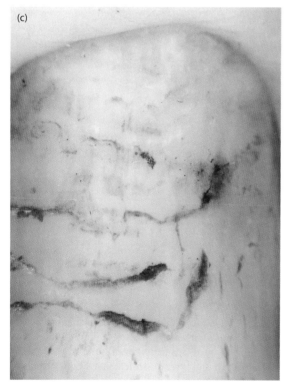

Figure 19.2 Nail plate dermoscopy in nail pigmentation from exogenous sources. Dermoscopy clearly shows that the proximal margin of the pigmentation follows the shape of the proximal nail fold (a), superficial scales from keratin degranulation are more stained from the pigment, which, in this patient, was due to a self-tanning lotion (b), and pigments also deposit into superficial grooves (c).

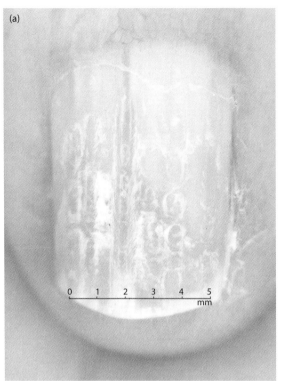

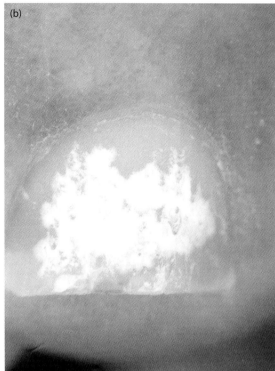

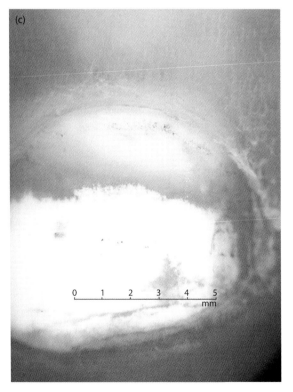

Figure 19.3 Nail plate dermoscopy in leukonychia. Dermoscopy easily distinguishes pseudo-leukonychia due to keratin degranulation (a) or white superficial onychomycosis (b) from true leukonychia (c), in which the nail plate surface is not affected.

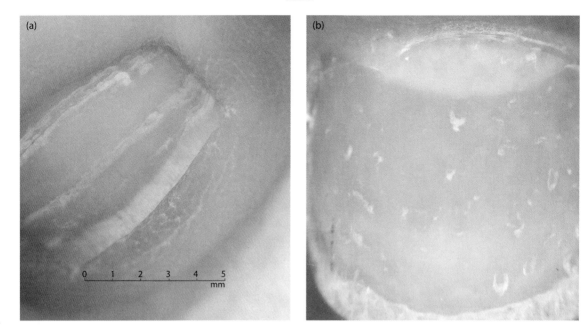

Figure 19.4 Nail plate dermoscopy enhances the visualization of nail plate surface abnormalities such as Beau's lines (a) and pits (b). Note the presence of desquamating cells on the pit surface.

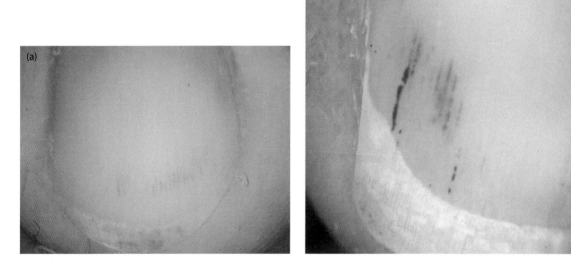

Figure 19.5 Nail plate dermoscopy enables visualization of nail bed vessels. Dilated vessels in the distal nail bed (a) and splinter hemorrhages (b) are commonly seen in nail psoriasis.

SUGGESTED READINGS

Lencastre A, Lamas A, Sá D, Tosti A. Onychoscopy. *Clin Dermatol.* 2013 Sep–Oct;31(5):587–93.

Piraccini BM, Bruni F, Starace M. Dermoscopy of nonskin cancer nail disorders. *Dermatol Ther.* 2012 Nov–Dec;25(6):594–602.

20 Dermoscopy of the proximal nail fold
Antonella Tosti

Examination of the proximal nail fold can be performed with nonpolarized dermoscopy using water or alcohol as the interface solution. Polarized devices can also be utilized in this area.

Box 20.1 Dermoscopy of the Proximal Nail Fold (Figures 20.1 and 20.2)

- Connective tissue disorders: Capillary enlargement and loss
- Periungual pigmentation: Pseudo-Hutchinson's versus Hutchinson's signs

---

Proximal nail fold dermoscopy is very important in the diagnosis and follow-up of connective tissue disorders.

In normal conditions, the proximal nail fold capillaries flow parallel to the skin surface and each capillary vessel resembles a hairpin, being formed by two arms that make a distal convex loop. They have a regular distribution, even with large intra/inter-individual variability. However, capillary loss and giant capillaries are not seen in the normal pattern. In connective tissue disorders, vessels are enlarged and tortuous and capillary loss with avascular areas is seen in dermatomyositis and scleroderma. The cuticle shows small hemorrhages and infarcts.

Dermoscopy is useful for evaluating pigmentation of the periungual tissues as it easily distinguishes the Hutchinson's sign from the pseudo-Hutchinson's sign, in which the cuticle looks pigmented as the underlying pigmentation is seen due to its transparency.

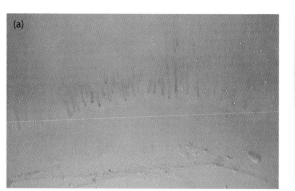

Figure 20.1 Dermoscopy of the proximal nail fold. In normal subjects, the proximal nail fold capillaries are uniform in morphology and are homogeneously distributed in small loops just above the cuticle (a). Giant capillaries are not seen in normal subjects; this patient has Raynaud's phenomenon (b).

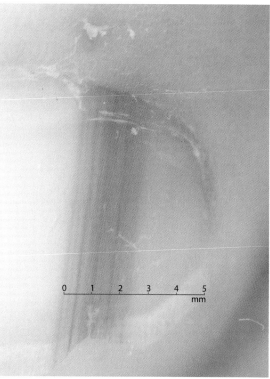

Figure 20.2 Dermoscopy of the proximal nail fold. The pigmented band is seen through the transparent cuticle (pseudo-Hutchinson's sign). This is seen even with pale bands.

SUGGESTED READINGS

Hasegawa M. Dermoscopy findings of nail fold capillaries in connective tissue diseases. *J Dermatol.* 2011 Jan;38(1):66–70.

Muroi E, Hara T, Yanaba K, Ogawa F, Yoshizaki A, Takenaka M, Shimizu K, Sato S. A portable dermatoscope for easy, rapid examination of periungual nailfold capillary changes in patients with systemic sclerosis. *Rheumatol Int.* 2011 Dec;31(12):1601–6.

Ohtsuka T. Dermoscopic detection of nail fold capillary abnormality in patients with systemic sclerosis. *J Dermatol.* 2012 Apr;39(4):331–5.

Park JH, Lee DY, Cha HS, Koh EM. Handheld portable digital dermoscopy: Routine outpatient use for evaluating nail-fold capillary changes in autoimmune connective tissue diseases. *J Eur Acad Dermatol Venereol.* 2009 Feb;23(2):207.

Tosti A, Piraccini BM, de Farias DC. Dealing with melanonychia. *Semin Cutan Med Surg.* 2009 Mar;28(1):49–54.

21 Dermoscopy of the hyponychium
Antonella Tosti

Examination of the hyponychium can be performed using a water or alcohol solution. Polarized devices that do not require the application of immersion fluids can also be utilized in this area.

The simple architecture of the hyponychium capillary network makes capillary loops in this anatomic area appear as regular red dots because of their perpendicular arrangement to the skin (each observed red dot represents the top of one loop).

> *Box 21.1* Dermoscopy of the Hyponychium (Figures 21.1 and 21.2)
>
> • Hutchinson's sign versus pseudo-Hutchinson's sign
> • Vascular abnormalities in nail psoriasis

Use of dermoscopy in the hyponychium can detect:

The micro-Hutchinson's sign: This is pigmentation of the periungual tissue that could not be seen with the naked eye. This may be important for the early diagnosis of subungual melanoma. Dermoscopy can distinguish the "malignant" Hutchinson's sign from the "benign" Hutchinson's sign. In the "malignant" Hutchinson's sign, dermoscopy shows the parallel ridge pattern, characterized by accentuated pigmentation in the deep intermediate ridges, with or without obliteration of the eccrine gland ducts. In the "benign" Hutchinson's sign, dermoscopy shows a brushy linear pigmentation across the skin marks; this is commonly seen in the benign nevi of children.

Vascular abnormalities: In nail psoriasis, the vessels of the hyponychium are coiled and twisted.

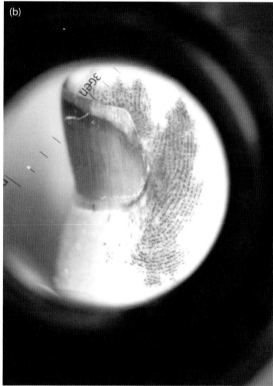

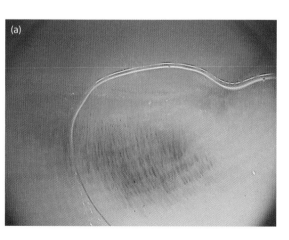

Figure 21.1 Benign Hutchinson's sign with brushy liner pigmentation (a) versus malignant Hutchinson's sign (b) with a parallel ridge pattern. (Courtesy of Elaine Siegfried, Saint Louis University, USA.)

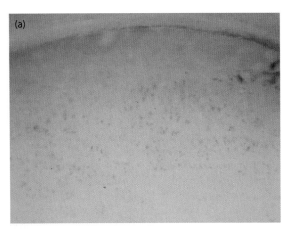
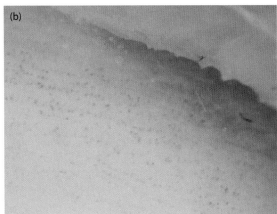

Figure 21.2 (a, b) Coiled twisted capillaries in nail psoriasis.

SUGGESTED READINGS

Iorizzo M, Dahdah M, Vincenzi C, Tosti A. Videodermoscopy of the hyponychium in nail bed psoriasis. *J Am Acad Dermatol*. 2008 Apr;58(4):714–5.

Lencastre A, Lamas A, Sá D, Tosti A. Onychoscopy. *Clin Dermatol*. 2013 Sep–Oct;31(5):587–93.

Tosti A, Piraccini BM, de Farias DC. Dealing with melanonychia. *Semin Cutan Med Surg*. 2009 Mar;28(1):49–54.

22 Dermoscopy of the distal edge of the nail plate
Antonella Tosti

Examination of the distal edge of the nail plate is much better performed using polarized instruments. When using nonpolarized dermoscopy, a gel or immersion oil can be used.

Box 22.1 Dermoscopy of the Distal Edge of the Nail Plate (Figures 22.1 through 22.3)

- Nail pigmentation: Ventral versus dorsal nail plate
- Onychopapilloma
- Onychomatricoma

Dermoscopy of the distal edge of the nail plate is very useful for localizing the pigment within the nail plate. This is important for understanding the site of melanin production as pigmentation in the ventral nail plate indicates that the lesion is localized in the distal nail matrix, whereas pigmentation in the dorsal nail plate indicates that the lesion is localized in the proximal nail matrix. Distal edge dermoscopy can then be used as a preoperative tool to select the anatomical site of excision.

Dermoscopy is also very important in the clinical diagnosis of nail tumors, such as onychopapilloma, in which it shows a focal keratotic mass underneath the free edge of the nail plate, or onychomatricoma, in which it shows multiple holes in the distal margin.

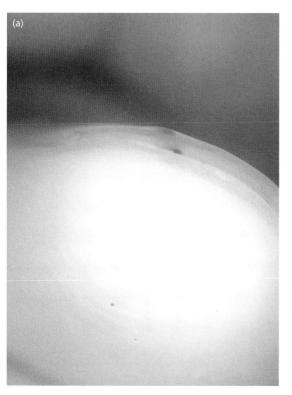
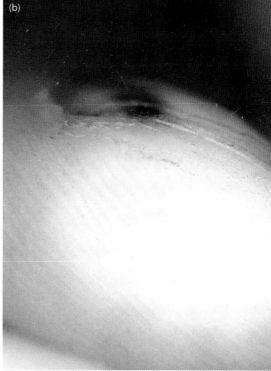

Figure 22.1 Dermoscopy of the distal edge of the nail plate enables the localization of the site of the pigmented lesion. Location in the ventral nail plate (a) indicates that the lesion is located in the distal matrix. When the pigment involves the entire nail thickness, the proximal matrix is also involved (b).

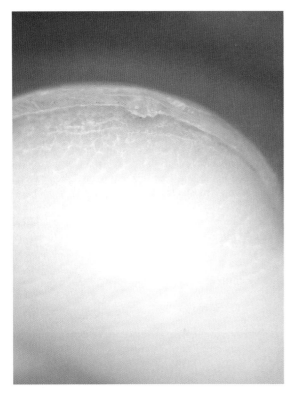

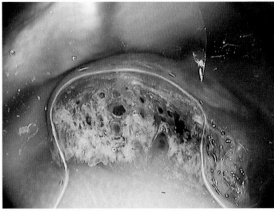

Figure 22.3 Onychomatricoma: the distal margin shows multiple holes with a woodworm appearance.

SUGGESTED READINGS

Braun RP, Baran R, Saurat JH, Thomas L. Surgical pearl: Dermoscopy of the free edge of the nail to determine the level of nail plate pigmentation and the location of its probable origin in the proximal or distal nail matrix. *J Am Acad Dermatol.* 2006 Sep;55(3):512–3.

Miteva M, Fanti PA, Romanelli P, Zaiac M, Tosti A. Onycho-papilloma presenting as longitudinal melanonychia. *J Am Acad Dermatol.* 2012 Jun;66(6):e242–3.

Figure 22.2 Onychopapilloma: note the keratotic mass at the free edge in correspondence with the band.

23 Inflammatory nail disorders
Antonella Tosti

NAIL PSORIASIS

Box 23.1 Nail Psoriasis (Figures 23.1 through 23.4)

- Pitting and other nail plate surface abnormalities
- Erythematous borders, oily spots, and splinter hemorrhages
- Twisted capillaries in the hyponychium

Nail plate surface abnormalities are better seen with polarized instruments. Psoriatic pits are large and irregular and dermoscopy shows the presence of scales around and within the pits.

Dermoscopy enables better visualization of the erythematous border that characterizes psoriatic onycholysis. Splinter hemorrhages appear as single or multiple red–brown linear or filamentous lines localized in the distal nail bed. Enlargement of the distal nail bed capillaries can also be seen.

Dermoscopy of the hyponychium is very useful for confirming the diagnosis of nail psoriasis in uncertain cases by showing irregularly distributed, dilated, tortuous, twisted capillaries, similar to those seen on the scalp. A magnification of 40× is needed for optimal visualization. Twisted, enlarged capillaries are also seen in Hallopeau's acrodermatitis.

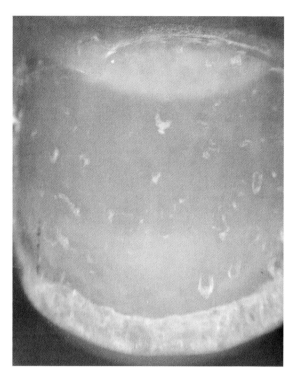

Figure 23.1 Nail psoriasis: psoriatic pits surrounded and/or covered by scales. Also note the splinter hemorrhages.

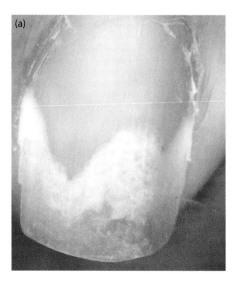
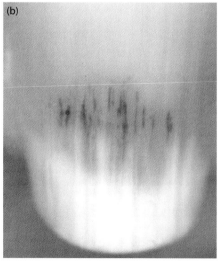

Figure 23.2 Nail psoriasis: dermoscopy enables the good visualization of the erythematous border in patients with onycholysis (a). Splinter hemorrhages are seen in the distal nail bed. They appear as fine red–brown lines of irregular thickness (b).

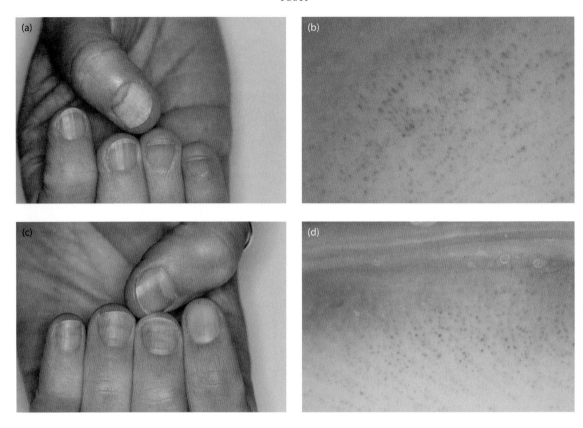

Figure 23.3 Nail psoriasis: in the patient with simple onycholysis due to nail psoriasis (a), dermoscopy enabled the diagnosis (b). In the patient with onycholysis with an erythematous border due to nail psoriasis (c), dermoscopy enabled the diagnosis (d).

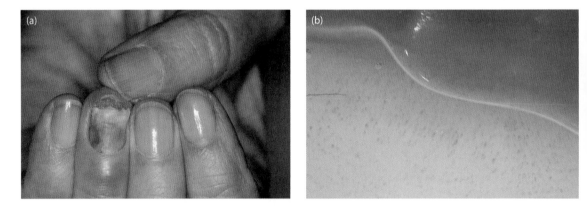

Figure 23.4 Hallopeau's acrodermatitis (a). Twisted, enlarged capillaries at dermoscopy (b).

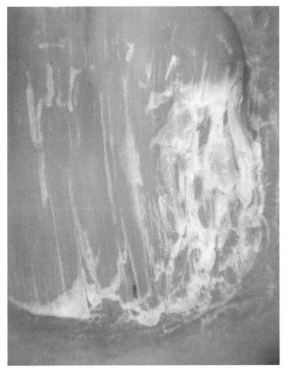

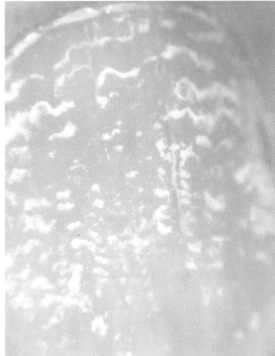

Figure 23.5 Nail lichen planus: longitudinal fissures are very evident at dermoscopy.

Figure 23.6 Alopecia areata: small regular pits covered and surrounded by scales.

NAIL LICHEN PLANUS

Box 23.2 Nail Lichen Planus (Figure 23.5)

- Fissures and other nail plate surface abnormalities
- Dorsal pterygium
- Nail atrophy and melanonychia
- Mottled lunula

Dermoscopy is only useful for the better visualization of nail plate fissures, nail fragmentation, and other nail plate surface abnormalities in lichen planus.

ALOPECIA AREATA

Box 23.3 Alopecia Areata (Figure 23.6)

- Small and regularly distributed pits
- Punctate leukonychia
- Twenty nail dystrophy
- Mottled lunula

In alopecia areata, dermoscopy enables the better visualization of the nail plate surface. Pits are the most common abnormality: they are small, regularly distributed, and surrounded by scales.

SUGGESTED READINGS

Farias DC, Tosti A, Chiacchio ND, Hirata SH. Dermoscopy in nail psoriasis. *An Bras Dermatol.* 2010 Jan–Feb;85(1):101–3.

Iorizzo M, Dahdah M, Vincenzi C, Tosti A. Video-dermoscopy of the hyponychium in nail bed psoriasis. *J Am Acad Dermatol.* 2008 Apr;58(4):714–5.

Lencastre A, Lamas A, Sá D, Tosti A. Onychoscopy. *Clin Dermatol.* 2013 Sep–Oct;31(5):587–93.

Nakamura R, Broce AA, Palencia DP, Ortiz NI, Leverone A. Dermatoscopy of nail lichen planus. *Int J Dermatol.* 2013 Jun;52(6):684–7.

Nakamura RC, Costa MC. Dermatoscopic findings in the most frequent onychopathies: Descriptive analysis of 500 cases. *Int J Dermatol.* 2012 Apr;51(4):483–5.

Piraccini BM, Bruni F, Starace M. Dermoscopy of non-skin cancer nail disorders. *Dermatol Ther.* 2012 Nov–Dec;25(6):594–602.

24 Traumatic nail disorders
Antonella Tosti

HEMATOMA

Subungual hematomas are common nail bed injuries caused by trauma to the fingers or toes. The affected nail shows a patchy or diffuse pigmentation that migrates distally with nail growth.

Hematoma does not exclude malignancy, as patients with melanoma of the nail unit may experience spontaneous bleeding.

Upon dermoscopy, the hematoma usually appears as a homogeneous area of black, brown, or red discoloration. The color depends on its duration, as hemoglobin is

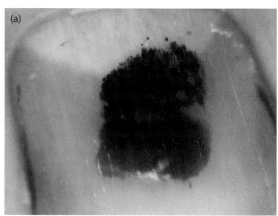

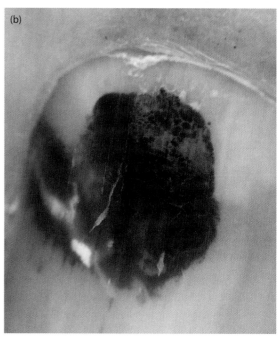

Figure 24.2 Subungual hematomas presenting as homogeneous areas of brown–purple discoloration. Diagnosis is indicated by the presence of peripheral round red spots (a) and a "filamentous" distal end (b). Also note the peripheral fading of the pigmentation.

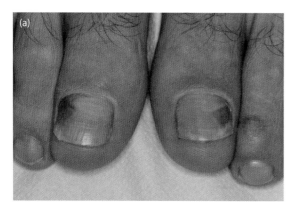

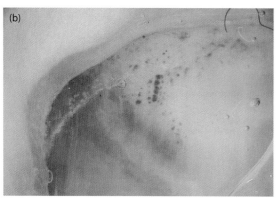

Figure 24.1 Subungual hematoma (a). Dermoscopy shows homogeneous red discoloration with round red spots at the periphery (b).

degraded by phagocytes into hemosiderin. The presence of red coloring in old lesions indicates a small amount of new bleeding, presumably due to repetitive trauma to the nail. The red and purple color components of the lesion are more evident with the dermatoscope. The presence of a "filamentous" distal end and/or round dark red spots at the periphery is very suggestive of this diagnosis. Peripheral fading and periungual or splinter hemorrhages are also commonly seen.

ONYCHOLYSIS

> *Box 24.2* Onycholysis (Figures 24.4 and 24.5)
>
> - Rollercoaster shape in the fingernails
> - Sharp proximal border in the toenails
> - Diagnosis suggested by the presence of round, dark red hemorrhagic spots and splinter hemorrhages

Traumatic onycholysis can involve the fingernails, which is most commonly occupational or induced by manicures, or the toenails of adults, which is usually caused by improper shoe wearing.

Dermoscopy often reveals round hemorrhagic spots or splinter hemorrhages that indicate the traumatic origin.

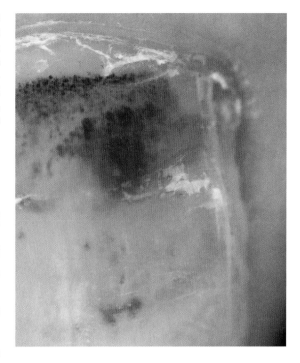

Figure 24.3 Subungual hematoma: the presence of round bright red spots at the periphery suggests recent bleeding.

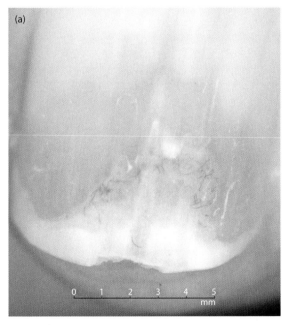

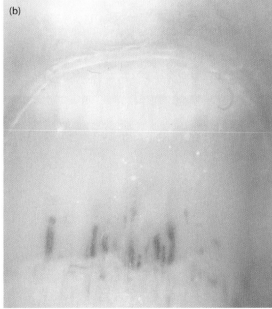

Figure 24.4 Traumatic onycholysis of the fingernails in a hairdresser. Dermoscopy shows hair fragments within the onycholytic space (a). This patient utilized a dental pick to clean her nails daily. Note the splinter hemorrhages at the border of the onycholytic area (b).

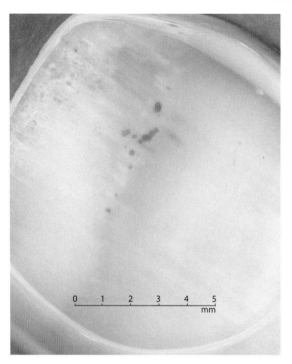

Figure 24.5 Traumatic onycholysis of the toenails: note the sharp proximal borders and round hemorrhagic spots within and around the onycholytic area.

TRAUMATIC LEUKONYCHIA

Box 24.3 Traumatic Leukonychia (Figure 24.6)

- Punctate or transverse true leukonychia
- Normal nail surface

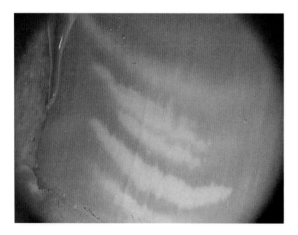

Figure 24.6 Transverse leukonychia of the big toe: the nail plate surface is normal.

Transverse leukonychia due to trauma can affect the fingernails, which is usually due to manicures, or the big toenails, which is due to the repetitive trauma to the distal edge of toenails from the tips of shoes. Dermoscopy shows white bands with a normal nail surface.

ONYCHOTILLOMANIA

Box 24.4 Onychotillomania (Figures 24.7 through 24.9)

- Hemorrhages of the nail bed and hemorrhages, crusts and scales of the periungual tissues
- Melanonychia
- Prominent vessels in the distal nail bed

Dermoscopic features of onychotillomania include scaling and crusts of the periungual folds associated with hemorrhages. When the nail plate is destroyed, the nail bed shows erosions and crusts.

Melanonychia due to melanocyte activation is common.

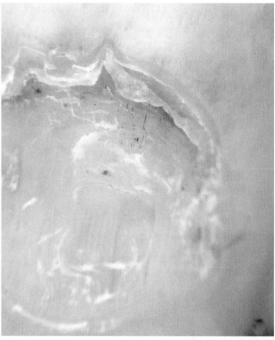

Figure 24.7 Onychotillomania: periungual crusting and scaling. The nail plate has been destroyed and the nail bed shows multiple splinter hemorrhages.

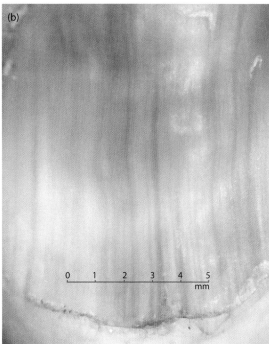

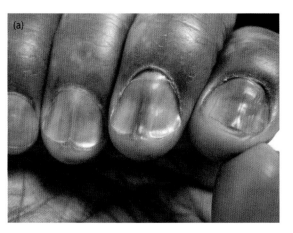

Figure 24.8 Onychotillomania: melanonychia, loss of the cuticle, and nail plate thinning and fissuring with koilonychia (a). Dermoscopy shows nail plate surface scaling and longitudinal brown–gray pigmented lines. Note that the lines appear to be on different planes due to the uneven nail plate (b).

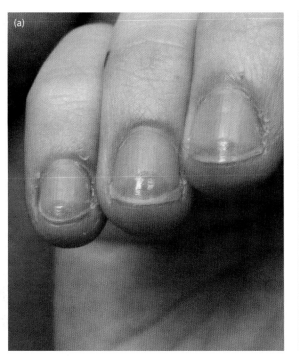

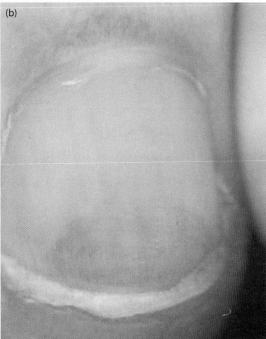

Figure 24.9 Onychotillomania: distal nail plate thinning due to excessive filing (a). Dermoscopy shows nail plate distal thinning with visualization of the nail bed capillaries (b).

SUGGESTED READINGS

Lencastre A, Lamas A, Sá D, Tosti A. Onychoscopy. *Clin Dermatol.* 2013 Sep–Oct;31(5):587–93.

Mun JH, Kim GW, Jwa SW, Song M, Kim HS, Ko HC, Kim BS, Kim MB. Dermoscopy of subungual haemorrhage: Its usefulness in differential diagnosis from nail-unit melanoma. *Br J Dermatol.* 2013 Jun;168(6):1224–9. Erratum in: *Br J Dermatol.* 2013 Sep;169(3):727.

Piraccini BM, Balestri R, Starace M, Rech G. Nail digital dermoscopy (onychoscopy) in the diagnosis of onychomycosis. *J Eur Acad Dermatol Venereol.* 2013 Apr;27(4):509–13.

25 Brittle nails
Antonella Tosti

Brittle nails are one of the most common nail complaints. Dermoscopy is useful for diagnosing pseudo-leukonychia due to keratin degranulation, in which the nail plate presents superficial desquamation. This is seen in women who continuously wear nail polish. Staining of the superficial scales is very common. In onychoschizia lamellina, dermoscopy shows that the distal nail plate desquamates in layers.

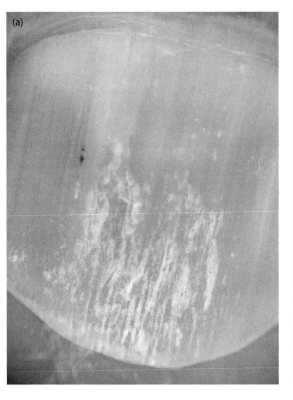 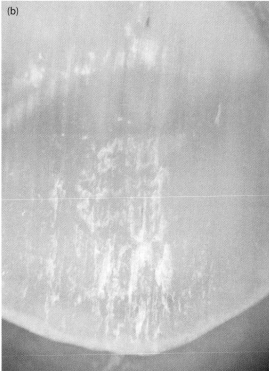

Figure 25.1 Pseudo-leukonychia from keratin degranulation: the whiteness is due to scales on the superficial nail plate (a, b). Scales may retain pigments from nail polish (c). *(Continued)*

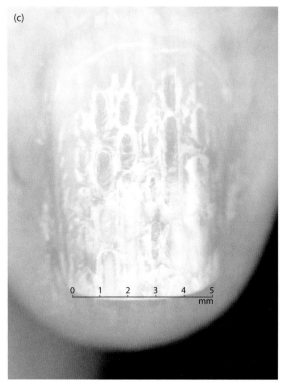

(c)

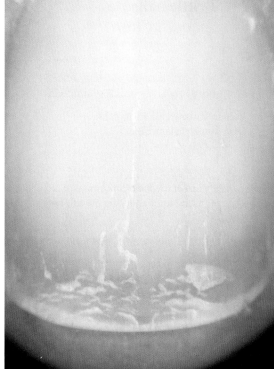

Figure 25.1 (*Continued*) Pseudo-leukonychia from keratin degranulation: the whiteness is due to scales on the superficial nail plate (a, b). Scales may retain pigments from nail polish (c).

Figure 25.2 Onychoschizia lamellina.

SUGGESTED READING

Herskovitz I, Nolan BV, Tosti A. Orange chromonychia due to dihydroxyacetone. *Dermatitis.* 2014 Jan–Feb; 25(1):43–4.

26 Onychomycosis
Antonella Tosti

Different clinical patterns of infection depend on the way and the extent by which fungi colonize the nail:

- In distal subungual onychomycosis, which is the most common type, fungi reach the nail from the hyponychium and colonize the nail bed.
- In proximal subungual onychomycosis, fungi penetrate the nail matrix via the proximal nail fold and colonize the deep portion of the proximal nail plate.
- In white superficial onychomycosis, fungi are localized on the nail plate surface.

Some fungi can produce melanin and cause nail pigmentation.

In distal subungual onychomycosis, dermoscopy shows that the onycholytic area has a jagged proximal edge with

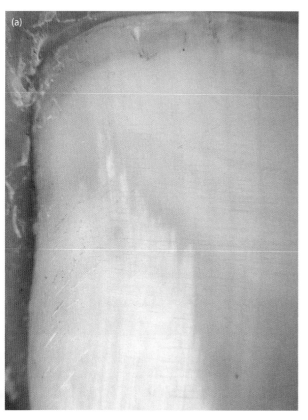
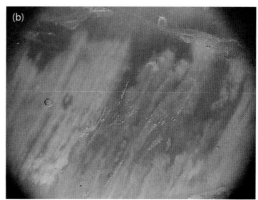
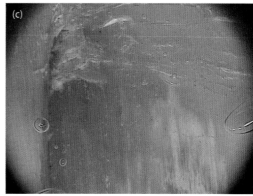

Figure 26.1 (a–c) Distal subungual onychomycosis: dermoscopy shows that the onycholytic area has a jagged proximal edge.

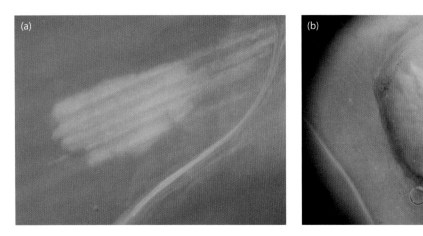

Figure 26.2 Distal subungual onychomycosis: dermoscopy helps with assessing severity by showing a patch corresponding to a dermatophytoma (a) or the involvement of the matrix area (b).

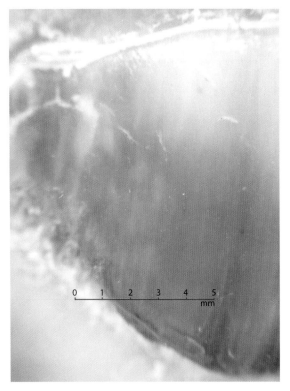

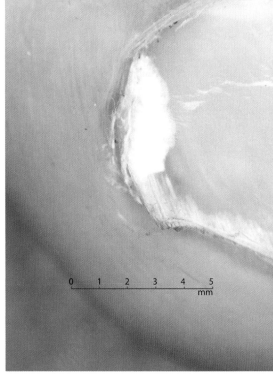

Figure 26.3 Pigmented distal subungual onychomycosis: dermoscopy shows the yellow streaks that suggest the diagnosis.

Figure 26.4 Proximal subungual onychomycosis: dermoscopy shows a patch of true leukonychia (the nail plate surface is normal) emerging from the proximal nail fold.

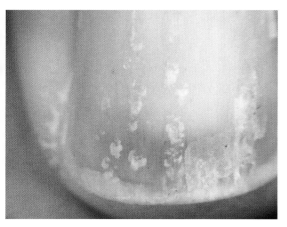

Figure 26.5 White superficial onychomycosis: dermoscopy shows pseudo-leukonychia; patches may have a yellow hue.

spikes. This pattern has been described as the "aurora borealis" pattern. It also shows longitudinal white–yellow streaks and patches and is useful for better delimiting the proximal progression of the infections.

In cases of pigmented onychomycosis, dermoscopy is very useful as it shows yellow streaks within the brown–black discoloration.

SUGGESTED READINGS

De Crignis G, Valgas N, Rezende P, Leverone A, Nakamura R. Dermatoscopy of onychomycosis. *Int J Dermatol.* 2014 Feb;53(2):e97–9.

Piraccini BM, Balestri R, Starace M, Rech G. Nail digital dermoscopy (onychoscopy) in the diagnosis of onychomycosis. *J Eur Acad Dermatol Venereol.* 2013 Apr;27(4):509–13.

27 Nail tumors
Antonella Tosti

Dermoscopy is very useful in the diagnosis of onychomatricoma and onychopapilloma, in which the observation of nail plate margin offers clues to diagnosis. In other tumors, dermoscopy may or may not provide diagnostic information.

Box 27.1 Nail Tumors

- Onychomatricoma
- Onychopapilloma
- Glomus tumor
- Myxoid cyst
- Fibroma/fibrokeratoma
- Warts
- Pyogenic granuloma
- Bowen/squamous cell carcinoma

ONYCHOMATRICOMA

Box 27.2 Onychomatricoma (Figures 27.1 and 27.2)

- Benign nail matrix tumor that develops within the nail plate.
- Longitudinal thickening and xanthonychia.
- Dermoscopy: Longitudinal white lines, proximal splinter hemorrhages, and distal splinter hemorrhages.
- Dermoscopy of the distal edge: Woodworm-like cavities.

Onychomatricoma is a benign tumor of the nail matrix that develops within the nail plate. The nail shows a band of longitudinal thickening that frequently has a yellow

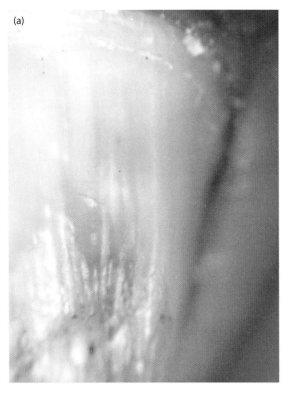
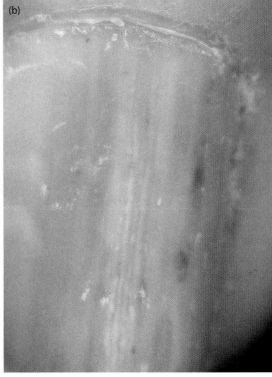

Figure 27.1 (a, b) Onychomatricoma: dermoscopy shows longitudinal white lines within the nail plate. Also note the yellowish color of the nail plate and splinter hemorrhages.

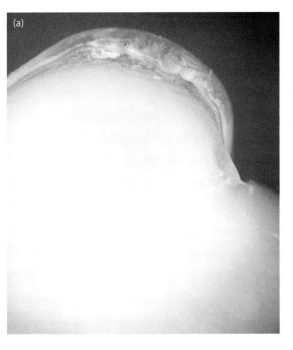

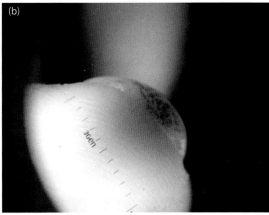

Figure 27.2 (a, b) Onychomatricoma: frontal view showing multiple holes with a woodworm-like appearance.

color. Multiple splinter hemorrhages are typical and often involve the proximal nail plate.

Nail plate dermoscopy shows longitudinal white lines that correspond to the channels that contain the tumor projections. The proximal and/or distal nail has multiple purple-to-brown splinter hemorrhages. Dermoscopy of the distal edge of the nail plate is often diagnostic, showing small woodworm-like cavities within the nail plate.

ONYCHOPAPILLOMA

Box 27.3 Onychopapilloma (Figure 27.3)

- Benign neoplasm of the distal matrix and the nail bed
- Longitudinal erythronychia, leukonychia, and melanonychia
- Dermoscopy: Single or multiple splinter hemorrhages within the band
- Dermoscopy of the distal edge: Subungual keratotic mass

Onychopapilloma is a benign neoplasm of the distal matrix and the nail bed.

Onychopapilloma is clinically characterized by longitudinal erythronychia, leukonychia, or melanonychia associated with hemorrhagic longitudinal lines.

The frontal view of the digit shows the presence of a small keratinized mass that adheres to the undersurface of the nail plate in correspondence with the band. The distal nail plate may present longitudinal splitting. Nail plate dermoscopy shows a homogeneous, pale red or whitish longitudinal band extending from the proximal nail fold to the distal edge. The proximal border of the band has a characteristic convex shape and its distal part may appear white because of onycholysis. In patients with dark skin, the band has a brown color. It contains one or more longitudinal, dark red-to-black streaks that correspond to splinter hemorrhages.

Dermoscopy of the distal edge of the nail plate shows a subungual keratotic mass that may contain hemorrhagic vessels.

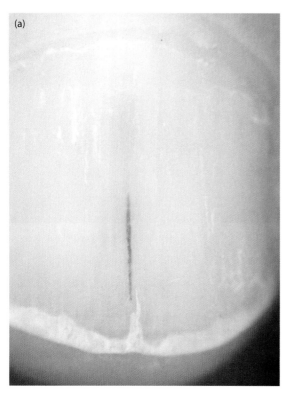

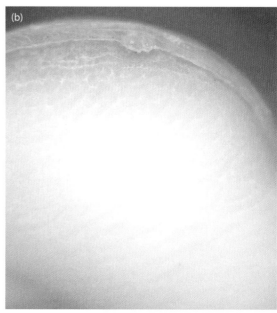

Figure 27.3 Onychopapilloma: homogeneous, pale red, longitudinal band with a convex proximal border. Note the splinter hemorrhage within the band (a). Frontal view revealing a typical keratotic mass under the affected nail plate (b).

GLOMUS TUMOR (FIGURE 27.4)

Dermoscopy may help with detecting subclinical lesions as irregular red–purple spots or linear vascular structures.

MYXOID CYST (FIGURE 27.5)

Dermoscopy can help with visualizing the nail plate groove and the connection to the proximal nail fold.

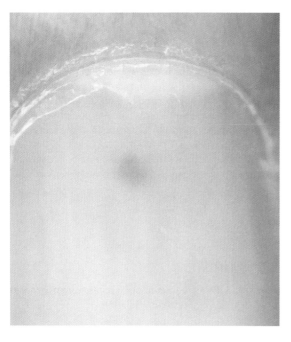

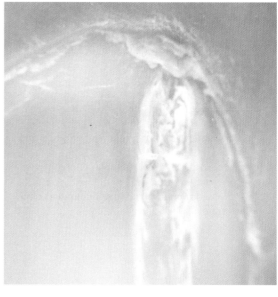

Figure 27.5 Myxoid cyst: irregular grooves and keratotic plugs on the proximal nail fold in correspondence with the cyst opening.

Figure 27.4 Glomus tumor visible as a small red patch.

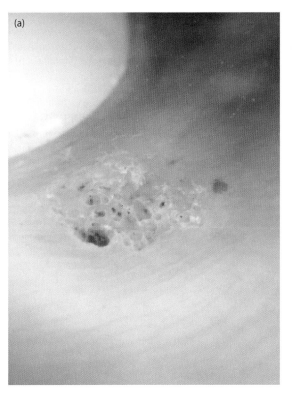
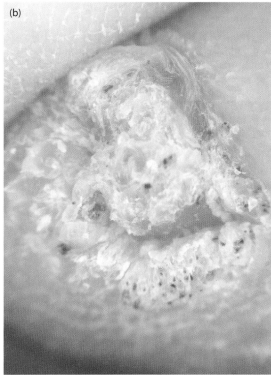

Figure 27.6 (a, b) Warts: the keratotic lesion contains numerous black dots. In large longstanding lesions, a biopsy should be done to exclude squamous cell carcinoma, even if dermoscopy shows the typical black dots (b).

FIBROMA/FIBROKERATOMA
Dermoscopy is not superior to clinical examination.

WARTS (FIGURE 27.6)
As with skin sites, dermoscopy shows black dots corresponding to vessels within the keratotic lesion.

PYOGENIC GRANULOMA (FIGURE 27.7)
The dermoscopic examination of the lesion shows a reddish homogeneous area that often presents a white collarette at the periphery. White lines similar to a double rail may intersect older lesions.

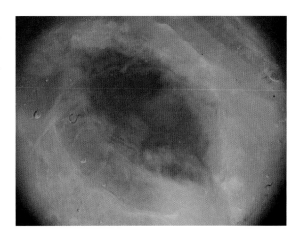

Figure 27.7 Pyogenic granuloma: reddish homogeneous area with a peripheral white collarette.

BOWEN'S DISEASE/SQUAMOUS CELL CARCINOMA (FIGURE 27.8)

In Bowen's disease, dermoscopy shows dotted vessels, islands of scales and hyperkeratotic, targetoid structures. White circles can be seen in squamous cell carcinoma.

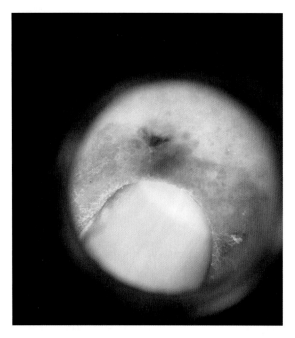

Figure 27.8 Bowen's disease: islands of scales and hyperkeratotic, targetoid structures. (Courtesy of Dr. Di Chiacchio, Brazil.)

SUGGESTED READINGS

Giacomel J, Lallas A, Zalaudek I, Argenziano G. Periungual Bowen disease mimicking chronic paronychia and diagnosed by dermoscopy. *J Am Acad Dermatol.* 2014 Sep;71(3):e65–7.

Lencastre A, Lamas A, Sá D, Tosti A. Onychoscopy. *Clin Dermatol.* 2013 Sep–Oct;31(5):587–93.

Maehara Lde S, Ohe EM, Enokihara MY, Michalany NS, Yamada S, Hirata SH. Diagnosis of glomus tumor by nail bed and matrix dermoscopy. *An Bras Dermatol.* 2010 Mar–Apr;85(2):236–8.

Miteva M, de Farias DC, Zaiac M, Romanelli P, Tosti A. Nail clipping diagnosis of onychomatricoma. *Arch Dermatol.* 2011 Sep;147(9):1117–8.

Miteva M, Fanti PA, Romanelli P, Zaiac M, Tosti A. Onychopapilloma presenting as longitudinal melanonychia. *J Am Acad Dermatol.* 2012 Jun;66(6):e242–3.

28   Melanonychia
Antonella Tosti

The term "melanonychia" describes the presence of melanin in the nail plate. Melanonychia most commonly appears as a longitudinal brown-to-black band of nail pigmentation, known as longitudinal melanonychia (LM). Transverse melanonychia can also occur. Pigmented lesions in the nail bed do not cause LM and are viewed through the nail as grayish-brown or black spots.

Nail pigmentation may be caused by melanocyte activation or by benign or malignant melanocyte hyperplasia. Melanonychia can be the first symptom of nail melanoma.

MELANOCYTE ACTIVATION

Melanonychia due to melanocyte activation is acquired, usually develops in adults and, in most cases, affects several nails. Causes of nail matrix melanocyte activation include dark phototype (racial melanonychia), drugs and

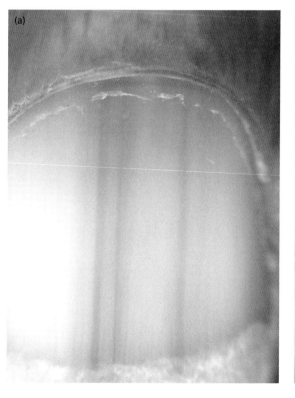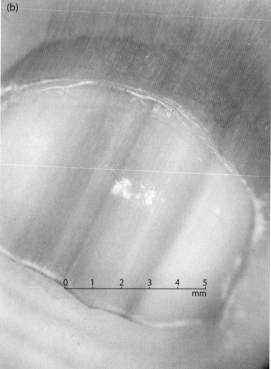

Figure 28.1 (a, b) Racial melanonychia: the bands are gray in color.

(a)

(b)

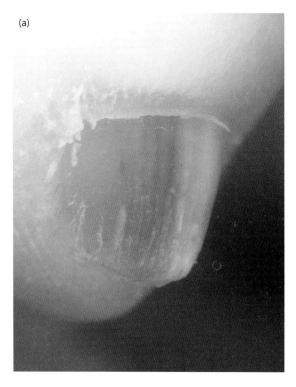
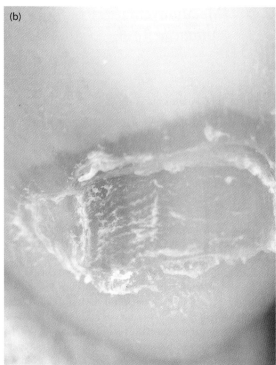

Figure 28.2 (a, b) Frictional melanonychia: gray band with small hemorrhagic spots (a). Pale brown homogeneous band; note the nail plate surface abnormalities due to friction (b).

postinflammatory, traumatic, systemic, and neoplastic nail disorders. Transverse melanonychia is always due to melanocytic activation.

At dermoscopy, bands due to melanocyte activation have a grayish background. The color varies from light to dark gray and the band may be homogeneous or contain thin, gray, regular, longitudinal parallel lines.

In traumatic melanocyte activation, tiny dark red-to-brown spots due to splinter hemorrhages or nail plate surface abnormalities may also be seen.

NEVI

> *Box 28.3* Melanonychia due to Nevi (Figures 28.4 through 28.8)
>
> - Most common cause of melanonychia in children
> - Congenital/acquired
> - Brown–black pigmented band of variable width
> - Dermoscopy: Adults: brown–black bands, sharp lateral borders, and thin, regular, longitudinal parallel lines; children: brown–black bands, irregular lines of different colors and thicknesses, dots and globules and brushy pigmentation across skin marks

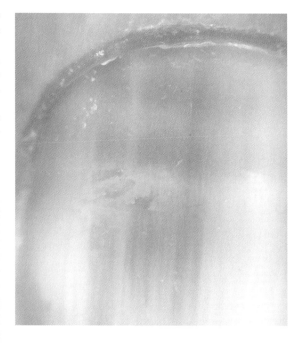

Figure 28.3 Drug-induced melanonychia in a patient undergoing chemotherapy. The color is gray and the pigmentation does not reach the distal nail.

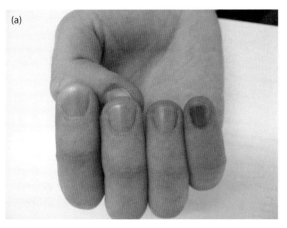

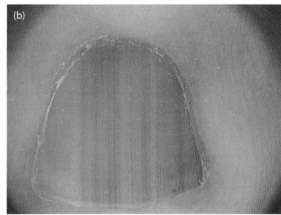

Figure 28.4 Nevus in a child (a). Brown band with regular lines (b).

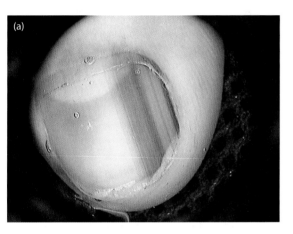

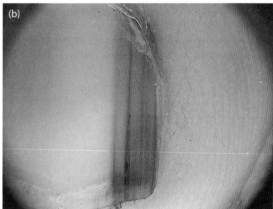

Figures 28.5 Nevi in children often cause bands with lines of irregular colors and thicknesses. Note the pseudo-Hutchinson's sign (a) and linear pigmentation across the skin marks in the hyponychium (b).

Nevi can be congenital or acquired. They are the most common cause of melanonychia in children. The nail presents one or more longitudinal pigmented bands varying in size from a few millimeters to the whole nail width and in color from light brown to black.

In adults, bands due to nail matrix nevi usually have sharply delimited lateral borders and contain thin, regular, longitudinal brown or black parallel lines. In children, the longitudinal lines are frequently irregular in color and thickness, the nail plate may contain dots and globules and the hyponychium can present brushy, linear pigmentation across the skin marks. Very dark bands are often associated with pigmentation of the cuticle due to the fact that the dark nail plate pigmentation is visible through the transparent nail fold. This is referred to as the pseudo-Hutchinson's sign and is not a sign of malignancy.

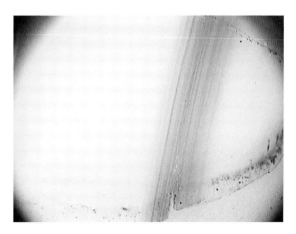

Figure 28.6 Nevus in a 7-year-old child: brown band with a homogeneous line but splitting of the distal nail plate.

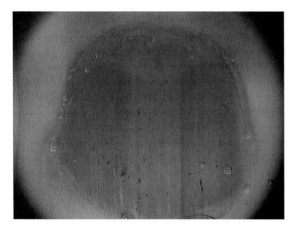

Figure 28.7 Nevus in a child: homogeneous brown band with melanin granules.

MELANOMA

Box 28.4 Melanonychia due to Nail Matrix Melanoma (Figures 28.9 through 28.14)

- Usually seen in adults
- Most commonly of the thumb/big toe
- Brown–black pigmented band of variable width (70% of cases)
- Pigmentation of the nail fold/hyponychium (Hutchinson's sign)
- Dermoscopy: Blurred lateral margin, longitudinal lines of different thicknesses and colors with disruption of parallelism, very dark homogeneous pigmentation, and parallel ridge pattern in the hyponychium

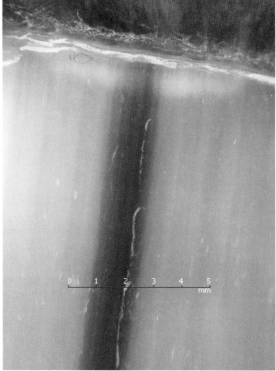

Figure 28.8 Nevus in a 4-year-old black child: black homogeneous band with blurred margins.

Nail matrix melanoma usually presents as a band of LM.

The nail plate may present a fissure or a split in correspondence with the band, indicating compression or destruction of the nail matrix epithelium by the melanoma.

(a)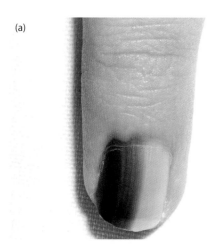

(b)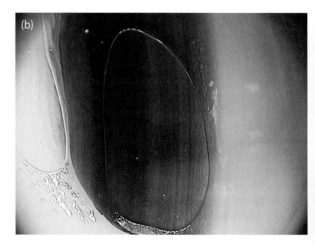

Figure 28.9 Nail melanoma "*in situ*" (a). Dermoscopy shows a dark brown band with lines of irregular colors and thicknesses (b).

Bands due to nail matrix melanoma have blurred lateral margins and contain longitudinal lines of different thicknesses and colors with disruption of parallelism. It is quite common to see very dark bands without visible lines. Pigmentation of the hyponychium shows the typical parallel ridge pattern seen in acral melanoma. Dermoscopy is also useful for detecting the micro-Hutchinson's sign on the cuticle or on the hyponychium.

Amelanotic melanoma represents approximately 25% of nail melanomas. Dermoscopy shows atypical vascularity and focal irregular remnants of pigmentation. Polymorphic vascular structures include milky-red areas, irregular linear vessels, hairpin vessels, and dotted vessels.

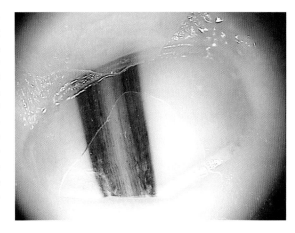

Figure 28.10 Nail melanoma: the band has a triangular shape and irregular lines of different colors and thicknesses. Also note the melanin granules.

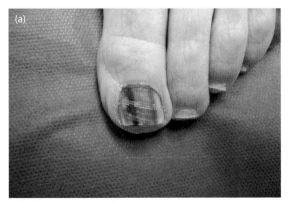

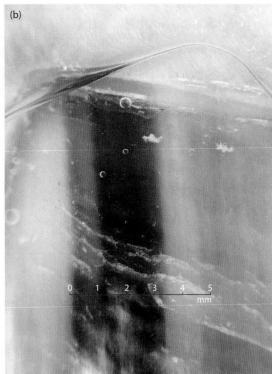

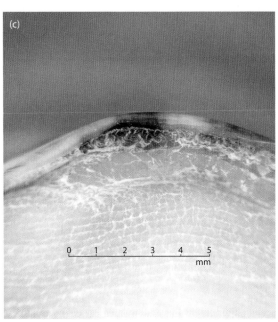

Figure 28.11 Nail melanoma (a). Dark black band without visible lines, and the surrounding nail plate shows a diffuse gray-to-brown pigmentation (b). The frontal view shows that the pigmentation involves the whole nail thickness, although it is more pronounced on ventral nail plate (c).

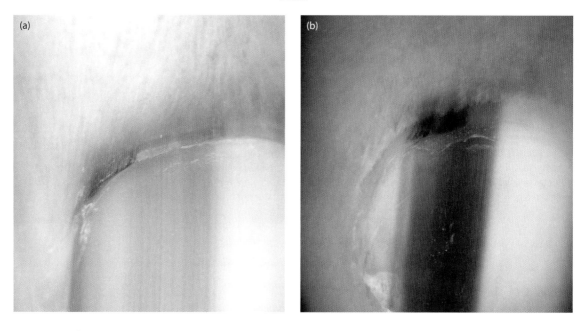

Figure 28.12 (a, b) Nail melanoma: microscopic Hutchinson's sign at the level of the cuticle. (Figure 28.12b is courtesy of Dr. Nilton Di Chiacchio, Brazil.)

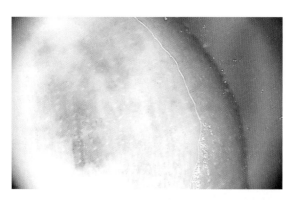

Figure 28.13 Hutchinson's sign of the hyponychium with a typical parallel ridge pattern.

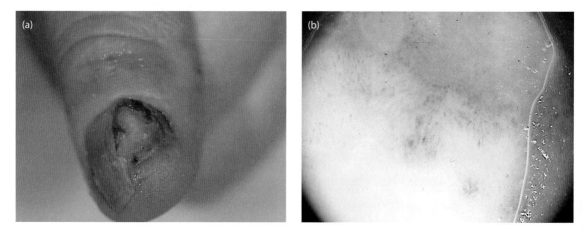

Figure 28.14 Amelanotic melanoma (a). Dermoscopy shows focal irregular remnants of pigmentation and atypical vascularity (b).

INTRAOPERATIVE DERMOSCOPY

Box 28.5 Intraoperative Dermoscopy (Figures 28.15 through 28.17)

- Performed during surgery after nail plate avulsion
- Enables direct visualization of the pigmented lesion
- Four possible patterns:
  - Regular gray pattern/melanocyte activation
  - Regular brown pattern/benign melanocytic hyperplasia
  - Regular brown pattern with globules or blotches/nevi
  - Irregular pattern/melanoma

Intraoperative dermoscopy examination is performed directly on the nail matrix and bed after nail plate avulsion. This procedure enables the direct visualization of the dermoscopic patterns of the pigmented lesion.

Four intraoperative dermoscopic patterns have been described:

The regular gray pattern, characterized by the presence of fine regular grayish lines, is seen in melanonychia due to melanocytic activation.

The regular brown pattern is associated with typical melanocytic hyperplasia.

The regular brown pattern with globules or blotches is associated with melanocytic nevi, where globules correspond to nests of nevus cells.

The irregular pattern is characterized by the presence of longitudinal lines of irregular colors and thicknesses, with or without irregular globules or blotches, and is associated with melanoma.

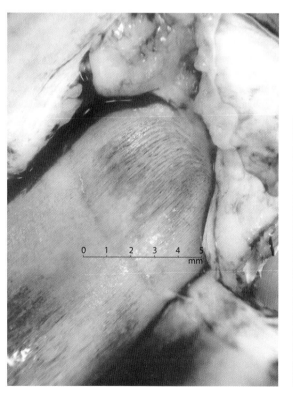

Figure 28.15 Nail lentigo: regular brown pattern.

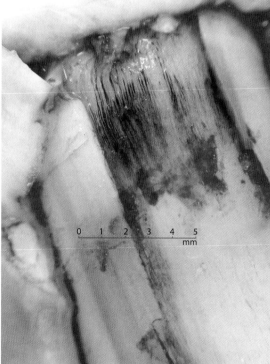

Figure 28.16 Nail melanoma: longitudinal lines of irregular thickness with irregular blotches.

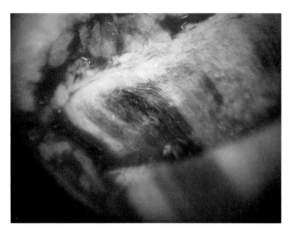

Figure 28.17 Nail melanoma: Intraoperative dermoscopy of the patient depicted in Figure 28.13. Irregular lines are visible. (Courtesy of Dr. Nilton Di Chiacchio, Brazil.)

SUGGESTED READINGS

Braun RP, Baran R, Saurat JH, Thomas L. Surgical Pearl: dermoscopy of the free edge of the nail to determine the level of nail plate pigmentation and the location of its probable origin in the proximal or distal nail matrix. *J Am Acad Dermatol.* 2006 Sep;55(3):512–3.

Di Chiacchio N, Hirata SH, Enokihara MY, Michalany NS, Fabbrocini G, Tosti A. Dermatologists' accuracy in early diagnosis of melanoma of the nail matrix. *Arch Dermatol.* 2010 Apr;146(4):382–7.

Di Chiacchio N, Ruben BS, Loureiro WR. Longitudinal melanonychias. *Clin Dermatol.* 2013 Sep–Oct; 31(5):594–601.

Di Chiacchio ND, Farias DC, Piraccini BM, Hirata SH, Richert B, Zaiac M, Daniel R et al. Consensus on melanonychia nail plate dermoscopy. *An Bras Dermatol.* 2013 Mar–Apr;88(2):309–13.

Hirata SH, Yamada S, Almeida FA, Tomomori-Yamashita J, Enokihara MY, Paschoal FM, Enokihara MM, Outi CM, Michalany NS. Dermoscopy of the nail bed and matrix to assess melanonychia striata. *J Am Acad Dermatol.* 2005 Nov;53(5):884–6.

Hirata SH, Yamada S, Enokihara MY, Di Chiacchio N, de Almeida FA, Enokihara MM, Michalany NS, Zaiac M, Tosti A. Patterns of nail matrix and bed of longitudinal melanonychia by intraoperative dermatoscopy. *J Am Acad Dermatol.* 2011 Aug;65(2):297–303.

Inoue Y, Menzies SW, Fukushima S, Nishi-Kogushi H, Miyashita A, Masukuchi S, Muchemwa F, Kageshita T, Ihn H. Dots/globules on dermoscopy in nail-apparatus melanoma. *Int J Dermatol.* 2014 Jan;53(1): 88–92

Mun JH, Kim GW, Jwa SW, Song M, Kim HS, Ko HC, Kim BS, Kim MB. Dermoscopy of subungual haemorrhage: Its usefulness in differential diagnosis from nail-unit melanoma. *Br J Dermatol.* 2013 Jun;168(6):1224–9. Erratum in: *Br J Dermatol.* 2013 Sep;169(3):727.

Phan A, Dalle S, Touzet S, Ronger-Savlé S, Balme B, Thomas L. Dermoscopic features of acral lentiginous melanoma in a large series of 110 cases in a white population. *Br J Dermatol.* 2010 Apr;162(4):765–71.

Ronger S, Touzet S, Ligeron C, Balme B, Viallard AM, Barrut D, Colin C, Thomas L. Dermoscopic examination of nail pigmentation. *Arch Dermatol.* 2002 Oct;138(10):1327–33.

Sawada M, Yokota K, Matsumoto T, Shibata S, Yasue S, Sakakibara A, Kono M, Akiyama M. Proposed classification of longitudinal melanonychia based on clinical and dermoscopic criteria. *Int J Dermatol.* 2014 May;53(5):581–5.

Thomas L, Phan A, Pralong P, Poulalhon N, Debarbieux S, Dalle S. Special locations dermoscopy: Facial, acral, and nail. *Dermatol Clin.* 2013 Oct;31(4):615–24.

Tosti A, Argenziano G. Dermoscopy allows better management of nail pigmentation. *Arch Dermatol.* 2002 Oct;138(10):1369–70.

Tosti A, Piraccini BM, de Farias DC. Dealing with melanonychia. *Semin Cutan Med Surg.* 2009 Mar;28(1): 49–54.

29 Connective tissue disorders
Antonella Tosti

Nail fold capillaroscopy is useful both as a diagnostic tool and as a predictor of disease progression.

Morphological changes in the nail fold capillaries confirm the diagnosis of autoimmune connective tissue diseases. The severity in the capillary changes has been related to systemic disease activity.

Magnifications of 30×–50× are usually utilized.

SCLERODERMA

In early scleroderma, proximal nail fold dermoscopy shows few enlarged/giant capillaries, few capillary hemorrhages, relatively well-preserved capillary distributions, and no evident loss of capillaries. In active disease, dermoscopy shows frequent giant capillaries, frequent capillary hemorrhages, moderate loss of capillaries, mild disorganization of the capillary architecture, and absent or mild ramified capillaries. In advanced disease, capillary enlargement is associated with a loss of capillaries with extensive avascular areas and disorganization of the normal capillary array with ramified/bushy capillaries.

Pterygium inversum unguis, also known as ventral pterygium, describes the adherence of the hyponychium to the ventral nail plate and is easily seen at dermoscopy.

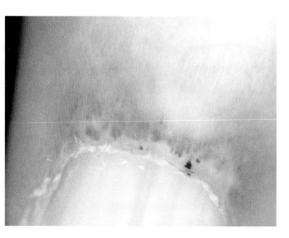

Figure 29.1 Active scleroderma: dermoscopy shows capillary loss and enlarged capillaries with hemorrhages.

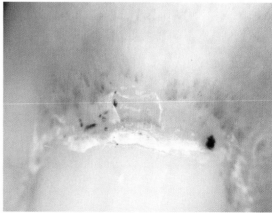

Figure 29.2 Advanced scleroderma: avascular areas and bushy capillaries.

195

DERMATOMYOSITIS

Box 29.3 Dermatomyositis (Figures 29.3 and 29.4)

- Capillary enlargement
- Capillary loss
- Cuticle hemorrhages

The dermatomyositis pattern is similar to the scleroderma pattern. Diagnosis of dermatomyositis is suggested by finding two or more of the following in at least two nail folds: enlargement of the capillary loops, loss of capillaries, disorganization of the normal distribution of capillaries, bushy capillaries, twisted enlarged capillaries, and capillary hemorrhages, often in the cuticle.

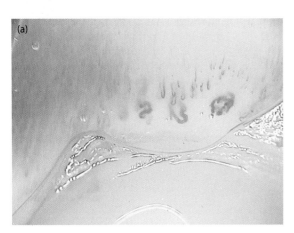
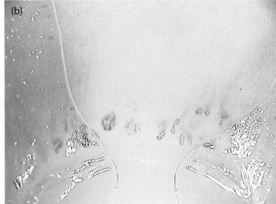

Figure 29.3 (a, b) Dermatomyositis: enlarged twisted capillaries and capillary loss.

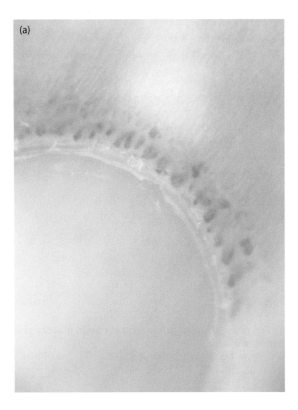
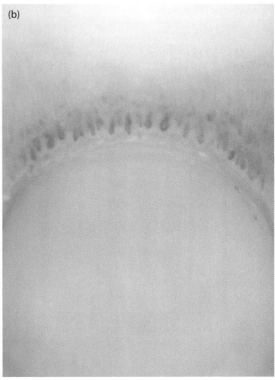

Figure 29.4 (a, b) Dermatomyositis: capillary enlargement and bushy capillaries.

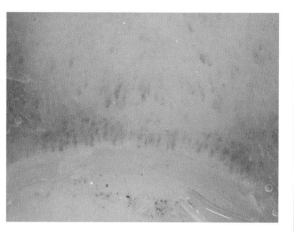

Figure 29.5 Systemic lupus erythematosus: enlarged tortuous capillaries and normal capillary density.

SYSTEMIC LUPUS ERYTHEMATOSUS

Box 29.4 Systemic Lupus Erythematosus (Figures 29.5 and 29.6)

- Capillary enlargement with dilated tortuous capillaries
- Normal capillary density

In systemic lupus erythematosus, the capillary density is normal but the capillaries are tortuous, elongated, and dilated.

SUGGESTED READINGS

Cutolo M, Sulli A, Secchi ME, Paolino S, Pizzorni C. Nail-fold capillaroscopy is useful for the diagnosis and follow-up of autoimmune rheumatic diseases. A future tool for the analysis of microvascular heart involvement? *Rheumatology (Oxford)*. 2006 Oct;45 (Suppl 4):iv43–6.

Hasegawa M. Dermoscopy findings of nail fold capillaries in connective tissue diseases. *J Dermatol.* 2011 Jan;38(1):66–70.

Muroi E, Hara T, Yanaba K, Ogawa F, Yoshizaki A, Takenaka M, Shimizu K, Sato S. A portable dermatoscope for easy, rapid examination of periungual nailfold capillary changes in patients with systemic sclerosis. *Rheumatol Int.* 2011 Dec;31(12):1601–6.

Ohtsuka T. Dermoscopic detection of nail fold capillary abnormality in patients with systemic sclerosis. *J Dermatol.* 2012 Apr;39(4):331–5.

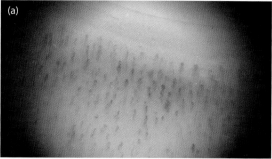

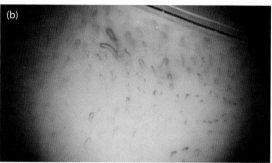

Figure 29.6 (a, b) Systemic lupus erythematosus: enlarged tortuous capillaries.

Index